DENIAL OF ILLNESS

Symbolic and Physiological Aspects

Publication Number 249
AMERICAN LECTURE SERIES®

A Monograph in
The BANNERSTONE DIVISION *of*
AMERICAN LECTURES IN NEUROLOGY

Edited by
CHARLES D. ARING, M.D.
Department of Neurology
University of Cincinnati College of Medicine
Cincinnati General Hospital
Cincinnati, Ohio

DENIAL OF ILLNESS

Symbolic and Physiological Aspects

By

EDWIN A. WEINSTEIN, M.D.

Associate Attending Neurologist
The Mount Sinai Hospital, New York
Consultant Neuropsychiatrist
Army Medical Service Graduate School
Washington, D.C.

and

ROBERT L. KAHN, Ph.D.

Research Psychologist
The Mount Sinai Hospital, New York

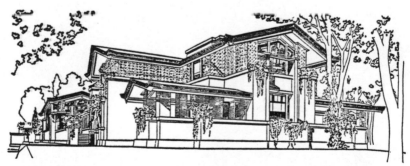

CHARLES C THOMAS • PUBLISHER
Springfield • Illinois • U.S.A.

CHARLES C THOMAS · PUBLISHER
BANNERSTONE HOUSE
301-327 East Lawrence Avenue, Springfield, Illinois, U.S.A.

Published simultaneously in the British Commonwealth of Nations by
BLACKWELL SCIENTIFIC PUBLICATIONS, LTD., OXFORD, ENGLAND

Published simultaneously in Canada by
THE RYERSON PRESS, TORONTO

Library of Congress Catalog Card Number: 55-6124

Printed in the United States of America

FOREWORD

THE PRESENT monograph represents the culmination of studies begun in 1938. At that time, under the stimulus of Dr. Sidney Tarachow, interest was centered in the amnestic-confabulatory state. The more intensive and systematic phase of the work has been going on since 1947. In the course of time, with the accumulation of data, certain of the earlier hypotheses were rejected as inadequate. It was gradually recognized that the motivation to deny illness provided a unifying concept to cover various patterns of behavior observed in altered states of brain function. ·

We are indebted to the many people who assisted us in various phases of our work, especially Drs. Louis Linn, Sidney Malitz, Jules Rozanski, Benno Schlesinger, Walter Slote, Hans Strauss and Leroy A. Sugarman. We are grateful to Dr. Israel S. Wechsler, Consulting Neurologist of The Mount Sinai Hospital, New York, Dr. Morris B. Bender, Attending Neurologist of The Mount Sinai Hospital, and Dr. David McK. Rioch, Technical Director, Neuropsychiatry Division, Army Medical Service Graduate School, for their cooperation and advice. We wish to thank the staff of the Neurological and Neurosurgical Services of The Mount Sinai and Walter Reed Army Hospitals for their help, and Mrs. Banda and Misses Skarulis and Ellis for deciphering and typing the manuscripts. The study has been supported in part by a grant from the Medical Research and Development Board, Office of the Surgeon General, contract no. DA-49-007-MD-376, the Neurological Research Fund of The Mount Sinai Hospital, and a grant-in-aid from the Lilly Research Laboratories.

E. A. W. and R. L. K.

CONTENTS

vii

DENIAL OF ILLNESS

Symbolic and Physiological Aspects

Chapter I

BACKGROUND AND STATEMENT OF THE PROBLEM

S TUDIES of denial of illness in the literature have concerned mainly cases of blindness and hemiplegia. While
denial of blindness has been called Anton's syndrome,
earlier cases were described by Von Monakow in 1885.
Since then a considerable number of additional cases have
been recorded.* While each patient had disease of the
brain, the blindness itself might result from a lesion anywhere in the optic pathway from the retina to the cal-
carine area. The patients either denied explicitly that they
were blind or spoke or acted in a manner indicating a lack
of recognition of the blindness. They described the surroundings in confabulatory fashion. When some awareness of the defect was expressed it was attributed to such
factors as "being in a dark cellar," "tears in my eyes" or
"not wearing my glasses."

The term "anosognosia" was introduced by Babinski in
1914 to denote denial or unawareness of left hemiplegia.
At a meeting of the Paris Neurological Society, Babinski
described the behavior of two such patients. One appeared

---

* Dejerine and Vialet (1893), Anton (1896), Rossolimo (1896),
Lunz (1897), Probst (1901), Mayer (1900), Raymond, Lejonne and
Galezowski (1906), Redlich and Bonvicini (1908), Albrecht (1918),
Pötzl (1924), Tunero (1931), Raney and Nielsen (1942), Weber
(1942), Goldstein (1939), Redlich and Dorsey (1945), Brockman and
Von Hagen (1946), Lutt (1947), Oppenheimer and Weissman (1951)
and Guthrie and Grossman (1952).

to have been unaware of the paralysis of her left limbs for several years. She would ignore commands to move her left hand. She never complained of her paralysis and never spoke about herself. The second patient stated that she was not paralyzed. When asked what her trouble was she gave "pain in the back" or "phlebitis" as the difficulty. When requested to move her left arm she either did not respond or said "Voilà, c'est fait." Both patients appeared to be clear mentally although Babinski stated that the psychic aspects had not been studied in detail. Subsequently both patients became demented. In discussing Babinski's paper, Souques described the behavior of a doctor with a left hemiplegia and hemianesthesia who had a "forgetfulness" of his left side and who, when the word "hemiparesis" was mentioned to him, seemed not to pay attention.

Subsequent reports similarly describe patients who verbally deny their paralysis and those who neglect and ignore the affected limbs. Critchley (1953), in a recent review of the literature, quotes accounts of other forms of anosognosia. Patients might ascribe the ownership of the paralyzed limbs to someone else, locate them out into space or otherwise detach them from the body or name the paralyzed members as other persons, animals or inanimate objects. Cases have also been described in which the patient expresses the delusion that there are multiple extremities on the paralyzed side. Usually the denial of the paralysis of the arm and hand is more prominent than delusions concerning the lower extremity.

Although etymologically the term anosognosia means "lack of knowledge of the existence of disease," it has been used largely to connote specifically the denial or unawareness of left hemiplegia. Many instances however, of anosognosia for other aspects of disease have been noted.

Several authors have reported denial of right hemiplegia.[*]
Stengel and Steele (1946) reported unawareness of
paraplegia. Lhermitte (1950) and Hamburg, Hamburg
and di Goza (1953) each observed a patient who denied
the absence of an amputated limb. Anton (1898) described
patients with deafness who claimed that they could hear.
Bonhoeffer (1903), studied a patient with alexia who
stated that he could read. N. Roth (1944) recorded denial of auditory agnosia and described the behavior of a
woman with hemiballismus who denied that she was having the abnormal movements even though she had bruised
herself. Fulton and Bailey (1929), Nielson and Raney
(1939), and Redlich and Dorsey (1945) observed patients who denied that they were ill at all or that they had
undergone operations.

Anosognosia for multiple disabilities has been noted frequently. The combination of anosognosia for both left
hemiplegia and blindness has been reported by Weber
(1942), Redlich and Dorsey (1945), Nielsen and Sult
(1939) and by N. Roth (1944). Patients with hemiplegia
may not only deny the paralysis of the limbs but also the
visual loss on the affected side. In commenting on Babinski's original presentation, Ballet told of patients with
brain tumors, who as the illness progresses stop complaining of headaches and affirm that they have no trouble in
vision after they become blind. A patient of Sandifer's
likewise denied both blindness and headaches. Ehrenwald (1930) made the interesting observation that a patient with anosognosia for hemiplegia also denied that she
was menstruating. Instances are also recorded in which

---

[*] Schilder (1932), Von Hagen and Ives (1937), Nielsen and Ives
(1937), Nielsen (1938), Olsen and Ruby (1941), Sandifer (1946),
Halloran (1946), Rosenbaum (1948), Nathanson, Bergman and Gordon (1952).

a patient with anosognosia for one disability denied others
as they developed. Redlich and Dorsey (1945) cited a
patient with diabetes and hypertensive retinopathy who
denied his blindness. Shortly after hospitalization he sustained a hemiplegia which he also denied. N. Roth (1944)
reported a case with consecutive anosognosia for blindness, auditory agnosia and left hemiplegia.

The preponderance of cases of left hemiplegia, however, has limited thinking about anosognosia to attempts
to explain only this particular phenomenon. Thus Babinski (1918) suggested that anosognosia might be peculiar
to lesions of the right hemisphere. Most of the discussion
in the literature has centered about the question whether
anosognosia is a unitary modality of dysfunction that is
produced by a focal lesion or whether it is an aspect of a
more generalized disturbance in brain function and behavior. The first view is expressed by Gerstmann (1942)
as "it (anosognosia) does not necessarily entail lowering
of general cortical or mental function. Indeed, the patients
are not as a rule demented. Their sensorium, orientation,
memory, attention and judgment are good except for the
amnestic-agnostic disturbance in the sphere of body
awareness and recognition. In other words, the activity
of the mind as a whole is uninterrupted."

Other writers believe that anosognosia is but one manifestation of a more widespread disturbance of function.
Thus Redlich and Bonvicini (1908) regarded denial of
blindness as not an agnostic defect but rather as a form
of Korsakoff syndrome occurring in a blind person. Redlich and Dorsey (1945) found evidence of diffuse cerebral pathology with disorientation, memory impairment
and confabulation in each of their six patients who denied
blindness. Sandifer (1946) expressed the opinion that
denial of hemiplegia or of blindness could occur with
lesions anywhere in the nervous system if there were a

clouding of consciousness. Spillane (1942) pointed out that in most of the cases reported in the literature there is an initial period of confusion or coma.

The fact that anosognosia for hemiplegia is associated as a rule with sensory loss in the affected limbs has led some authors to consider the phenomenon as a result of deafferentation. Dejerine in discussing Babinski's paper thought that the loss of sensation was the important factor. However, it has been pointed out that many patients have profound sensory defects without production of anosognosia while others may neglect or deny the existence of a limb in which they apparently perceive stimuli.

Following the work of Head and Holmes (1911) and Pick (1908), anosognosia was considered by many as a disturbance of the "body scheme." The usual view was that there was a representation of a three-dimensional image of the body in the parietal lobe of the minor hemisphere, or in the thalamus or the connections between the two. Thus destruction of this area or portions of it were said to produce a loss of the image of that part of the body from the individual's awareness. Cobb (1947) states that "in amnesia for the limbs of one side . . . the patient loses these limbs from the body scheme and ignores them . . . it is a reliable symptom indicating a sub-cortical lesion in the parietal region."

Autopsy studies have not resolved the conflicting views. The cases described have been mainly these of vascular disease, infiltrating tumors and diffuse encephalopathic processes. Most have shown extensive pathology, often with multiple lesions. Pötzl (1924) stated that anosognosia for hemiplegia was due to the coincidence of lesions in the parietal lobe and thalamus. Most observers have agreed that deeply situated lesions are necessary for the existence of anosognosia. But others including Schilder (1932), Critchley (1953), Gerstmann (1942) and M. Roth

(1949) state that injury to the parietal cortex alone may cause a disruption of the body scheme and consequent anosognosia. Nielsen (1938) believes that superficial parietal lobe lesions produce an unawareness of the existence of the opposite limbs while denial of paralysis is associated with an interruption of the connections between the thalamus and the parietal lobe.

A more dynamic approach involving motivational factors has been taken by others. Schilder used the confusing term "organic repression" whereby the patient excluded the unpleasant facts of hemiplegia or blindness from consciousness. It is of interest that the relatives of Babinski's patients, as described in his first paper (1914), considered the delusion providential. They asked the doctors to avoid all questions that might disenchant the patients and trouble them in their peace. Goldstein (1939) saw in anosognosia a type of adaptation in which the more complete the defect the greater was the defense. He regarded the denial in itself as a psychological mechanism present in normal persons and thus not created by brain damage. Sandifer (1946) stressed the motivation of the patient to be well and interpreted denial of paralysis in terms of avoiding a "catastrophic reaction."

It is apparent that one's concept of anosognosia is determined by the types of cases observed and the particular methods of study used. The data in the literature are almost always in the form of case reports without systematic control observations. For example, authors who describe certain lesions as being associated with anosognosia have not studied the behavior of patients with similar lesions who do not express denial of illness. The effects of increased intracranial pressure and subarachnoid hemorrhage are not evaluated. Though the question of diffuse versus focal disturbances in brain function has been debated there have been few reports utilizing EEG records.

Many patients were apparently seen only briefly without continued observation. There are very few detailed psychological or psychometric examinations to evaluate the degree of mental impairment. Although motivational factors are mentioned, there are no systematic personality studies. With one exception there have been no attempts to produce anosognosia experimentally.

The present account of a large number of patients with various forms of anosognosia endeavors to employ more comprehensive and systematic methods of study. The conditions of brain function have been correlated with EEG records. Interviews have been carried out regularly over long periods of time so that patients' behavior may be compared at different stages of brain function which occur in the course of a disease process. Control studies have been carried out so that the behavior of patients with anosognosia could be compared with other patients with similar types of brain lesions. The pre-morbid personality has been systematically evaluated, psychological tests have been given, and an attempt has been made to produce the phenomena of anosognosia experimentally. Also, we have considered anosognosia in its relation to other types of behavioral changes associated with brain disease.

Chapter II

EXPLICIT VERBAL DENIAL

THE TERM anosognosia has been used to denote both explicit denial and unawareness of disabilities. For purposes of clarity the various types will be considered separately. Explicit verbal denial may be defined as the direct negation in words of the disability. This form of anosognosia was observed in 52 patients. Of these 11 denied the presence of a left hemiplegia, three of right hemiplegia, nine blindness or a marked visual defect, one paraparesis, one the loss of the left arm (amputation), one the loss of an eye, one ptosis, while two dysphasic patients denied having any difficulty in speech. One patient denied having involuntary movements in her right lower extremity. Twenty-nine patients denied that an operation, usually craniotomy, had been performed. Four patients who had received brain injuries denied that they had occurred. Thirteen patients denied having been incontinent of urine even though the evidence was usually obvious. Three patients denied being incontinent of feces. Five patients with marked memory defects denied that anything was wrong with their memory. Four patients denied having been sexually impotent. In addition to denying a specific disability, many patients refused to admit the fact of illness in general. Often patients with obvious headache would deny that they had pain and others denied having vomited. The clinical, neurological and pathological data are summarized in Table 1.

PATTERNS OF EXPLICIT VERBAL DENIAL

Although any one patient might deny illness in a num-

10

ber of ways, five main patterns could be distinguished.

1. **Complete Denial**—These patients denied totally that they were ill in any respect. Thus a blind person claimed that he could see and a paralyzed patient confabulated that he could move his limbs and walk without difficulty.

2. **Denial of Major Disability**—These patients denied their major incapacities but stressed some less threatening or minor or trivial aspect of illness. A patient with a hemiplegia denied the loss of function in his limbs but complained of constipation. A patient who had had a craniotomy denied this procedure and said that she had had an operation for a "slipped disc." Frequently benign procedures as tonsillectomy and appendectomy were substituted for a craniotomy.

3. **Minimization or Attribution to Some Benign Cause**— A patient with a left hemiplegia said he could move his arm but was too "lazy" to do so. A patient attributed difficulty in using a paralyzed limb to its being "sore from injections." Another woman with a left hemiplegia remarked that "everyone's left side is weaker than the right." A patient with a loss of memory commented that "everyone forgets now and then." Patients following craniotomy attributed the bandages to a "sore throat" and "keeping warm" or said that the head has been shaven to "keep cool."

4. **Projection of Disability Outside of the Self**—Patients with hemiplegia said the paralyzed limbs did not belong to them, often attributing their ownership to the nurse or doctor. A woman with a history of severe headache associated with subarachnoid bleeding said that her husband was suffering from headaches. A patient with a third ventricle tumor brought to a doctor's office because of the symptoms of headache and failing vision requested that her daughters be examined as it was they who were ill. Three patients with hemiplegia displaced the paralyzed

arm into space, one stating that her right arm was lying on her bedside table "like a set of false teeth."

5. Temporal Displacement of the Disability—Patients stated that the illness or disability had existed in the past but that they were quite recovered now. Others with complete hemiplegia insisted that they would be able to walk within the next few days.

The successive use of various patterns of explicit verbal denial is illustrated in the behavior of the following patient:

Case 23

A 35-year-old woman was admitted to The Mount Sinai Hospital on September 21, 1951. After delivery of a 7-months-old fetus that died, she had developed pneumonia and a pelvic and bladder infection followed by a left hemiplegia. When interviewed for the first time on October 4, she denied that there was anything wrong with her left arm and said that she had come to the hospital because she was sick to her stomach "if you can call that being sick." When asked to move the left arm she claimed that she was doing so. The patient also stated that she had not lost her baby but had given birth to twins. She also denied having had a pelvic infection although an indwelling catheter was present. In the next interview two days later, the patient again stated that there was nothing wrong with her left arm, that she had been moving it all that day. When she was asked to raise it she said that it might belong to a doctor or another patient. Two days later she admitted that the left arm was "a little stiff and weak from rheumatism." In the same interview she identified the left arm as her daughter (aged 7), addressed it affectionately and remarked, "All our family are small." In an interview five days later, she answered most questions about her ability to move her left limbs by complaining of pain in her right arm. She claimed that the reason that she could not move her left

arm was that it was tied down. (The patient's right arm
was restrained because she would pull at the tubing of
her catheter.)

During the next few interviews the patient would remark in a bantering way that she could move her arm
when the doctors weren't about but not when they came
in. She began to move her left lower extremity and on
October 23 tried to walk with support. She became very
agitated over the weakness of her leg, talked of becoming
a cripple but took no notice of her still completely paralyzed left arm. During the next two to three weeks the
patient expressed direct denial only intermittently. She
would answer questions about her left arm with humorous
evasions and clichés as "just when you want it to do something it won't," "just needs a little practice," "come back
some other day, you bad man," and "would you mind if
I used my right arm instead?" On November 16 the patient, while admitting that the left arm was paralyzed,
confabulated that she had moved it earlier in the day.
During the interview she claimed that the arm was lying
on the bureau in her room.

In subsequent interviews the patient admitted her
paralysis, stating that she was sure she would be able to
move the arm in a few days. During the last two weeks
in which she denied her paralysis in interviews with doctors, she would admit to her mother that she was unable
to use her arm. On one occasion she told her nurse, "I'm
fooling the doctors so I can go home."

DENIAL OF MULTIPLE ASPECTS OF ILLNESS

The denial usually included more than one aspect of
illness. Thus patients with anosognosia for hemiplegia or
blindness would also deny having had a craniotomy or
being incontinent of urine. One patient (Case 24) denied
difficulty in walking, visual defect, the fact that she had
had an operation and stated that her convulsive seizures
had been due to "hysteria." Case 25 entered the hospital

with a paraparesis. With the progression of her illness (brain stem neoplasm) she developed difficulty in breathing so that a tracheotomy was performed. She then denied not only the weakness in her legs but the fact that the tracheotomy tube had been inserted. A patient did not necessarily deny all his disabilities. In Case 3, the patient, following a craniotomy, denied the operation and the history of sexual impotence, but expressed awareness of a visual field defect. Other patients who had been impotent sexually did not deny it though showing anosognosia for other incapacities.

DENIAL IN RELATION TO CAUSE OF THE DISABILITY

Although all 52 patients with explicit verbal denial had demonstrable brain damage, the disability that was denied was not necessarily caused by a lesion of the nervous system. One patient who had sustained a brain injury and a traumatic amputation of the left arm, denied that he had lost the limb. Another man had had an eye enucleated many years previously for an infection. After suffering a head injury with a right hemiparesis he denied not only the weakness of his right limbs but the loss of the eye. This point was illustrated ingeniously by Guthrie and Grossman (1952) who found that a patient with anosognosia for a left hemiplegia also denied her inability to move her right arm when it was tied down with the patient blindfolded.

DENIAL OF OTHER STRESSFUL EXPERIENCES

Not only was there anosognosia for physical disabilities and other aspects of illness but patients commonly denied the existence of other personal problems and felt inadequacies in their life situation. Thus in Case 1, the patient denied not only hemiplegia but the pelvic infection and the death of her baby. The patient (Case 28) who denied having had a craniotomy and described her condition as "slipped disc" confabulated that her mother was still living. Actually her mother had died in giving birth to the patient. Some patients with unhappy marriages denied that they were married. Case 13 was an unsuccessful accountant who not only denied the fact that he had had a craniotomy and impaired memory, but boasted that he was "the best tax lawyer in New York City" and had "written half of the books on the subject." It was apparent that there existed an organization of function in which the patient denied anything that he felt was seriously wrong with him, whether physical disease, personal inadequacies or traumatic events in his life.

CONFABULATIONS

Confabulations were used to amplify the denial and to explain away obvious manifestations of illness. A man with a self-inflicted gunshot wound of the brain (Case 44) explained his hospitalization and the spherical skull depression by saying that he had "tripped over the cat and hit my head on a golf ball." The situation of being in the hospital was accounted for by stories of being employed there, visiting a friend or relative, having a baby, taking a rest, having a check-up and other comparatively innocuous explanations. Patients who were blind described the clothes and features of persons around them. A woman who had shot herself confabulated that another girl had been shot and also that her mother had been killed in an automobile accident. Another type of confabulation, observed less frequently than the others, did not deal directly with the denial of the overt defect but was rather related to what the patient felt was an inadequacy in his life situation. A young man was interviewed several days following a lumbar tap for a subarachnoid hemorrhage which he had apparently sustained in a fall downstairs. The year previously he had been discharged from the Army where he had had a sedentary job in the Aleutians. He confabulated that he had received the Congressional Medal of Honor for his exploits with Carlson's Raiders. On the day that he received a lumbar tap he stated that he had entered the hospital so that an operation could be performed for the removal of Japanese shrapnel from his back. A soldier who had sustained a head injury when his jeep overturned maintained that he had been shelled by the enemy while bringing in suspected spies. In cases of head injury who recovered such confabulations about the nature of the injury outlasted all other manifestations of disturbed behavior.

DURATION AND CONSTANCY OF DENIAL

Anosognosia was maintained in each patient for periods ranging from several days to one year. The denial persisted despite all logical argument and evidence to the contrary. Thus patients who denied having had a recent craniotomy were shown their shaven heads and operative scars in a mirror without changing their beliefs. One soldier (Case 29) denied for months after being shot through the head by enemy mortar fire, that he had been wounded. He refused even to accept a Purple Heart decoration. He appeared rational in all other respects but persistently refused to accept the fact of his injury. He explained the scar by a fabrication about developing a boil with an account of going on sick call and receiving treatment. He would answer attempts to convince him of the truth with the remark, "If I'd have been wounded I would have known it." Visual field defects were denied even after it was repeatedly demonstrated that the patient could not see objects and people on the defective side.

AMNESIA FOR THE PERIOD OF DENIAL

In patients who recovered to the extent that the degree of brain damage no longer sustained the anosognosia, there was an amnesia for most of the previously expressed denial. Most patients when interviewed later said they recalled little or nothing. In a few instances these were interpreted as dreams. There was rarely any understanding of the dynamics of the behavior when it was discussed later. Patients generally gave a superficial explanation or some rationalization. A patient who had confabulated she was pregnant (Case 33) said she had thought so because her abdomen was distended. A woman (Case 34) who had addressed all doctors as "Barney" said that she did this because she didn't know their last names. The patient who denied having received a head wound gave as his reason for giving up his delusion the fact that he had seen the defect on an x-ray. However, during the period of anosognosia the x-ray of his skull had repeatedly been shown to him.

ABSENCE OF ANXIETY

Patients with complete explicit denial were usually bland and affable during interviews. Fulton and Bailey (1929) aptly described the attitude of a group of patients with third ventricle tumors who denied they were ill as one of "fatuous equanimity." Outside of interviews, some patients might seem depressed and perplexed but became bland·and assured while being questioned. Some patients who seemed dull and distant during certain parts of the interview would appear animated while expressing their denial of illness. Even when repeatedly questioned about their disabilities they rarely became disturbed or agitated. There was a conspicuous absence of the "catastrophic reaction" both in interviews and in psychological testing situations, and no suicidal attempts were reported in any of the patients. Persistent questioning frequently served to reinforce the denial. Anxiety, in the ordinary clinical sense, was not present. Anosognosic patients seemed to maintain a serene faith that they were well which remained firm despite all disbelief by others. One patient, speaking of her paralyzed left arm, remarked, "I know maybe you didn't see it but I have a feeling it moves." Another in a similar situation acknowledged the logic of the examiner's opinions but insisted her arm moved because "I can see it and feel it." Another patient terminated a discussion about her claim that she could walk, even though paralyzed, with the comment "If you look it up in your books, doctor, you'll find cases like mine."

MOOD AND PSYCHOMOTOR ACTIVITY

Psychomotor activity was usually diminished. When sought for interviews patients often would be found lying in bed with closed eyes, though responding promptly when addressed. The expressions of denial and the confabulations were not as a rule made "spontaneously" but would be elicited by questioning. From the standpoint of hospital administration the patients in this group were generally well-behaved, accepting medication and submitting to procedures without protest. Urinary incontinence was frequent, occurring in 39 cases. Even if incontinence were not denied explicitly, patients appeared to disregard it, commonly lying in a wet bed without complaint.

Pronounced euphoric or manic behavior was uncommon and was much more frequently observed in patients with implicit forms of denial. Transient paranoid attitudes were common, occurring in 26 patients while a predominantly paranoid outlook in relation to illness was shown by seven patients. Thus a man with a subarachnoid hemorrhage (Case 30) attributed his headaches to having been pounded on the head by the doctors. In these seven patients the denial was not as complete. They were more restless, complaining about the food and medication. Alterations in sexual behavior (exposure, masturbation, sexual advances, delusions with a sexual content) were noted in five of the paranoid group but were inconspicuous in patients with complete verbal denial. Depressed attitudes were infrequent, with only two patients (Cases 31 and 32) being so characterized for any length of time.

The following case report is illustrative of the behavior of a patient with a paranoid form of denial.

Case 7

A 38-year-old housewife was admitted to The Mount Sinai Hospital on March 14, 1949 because of severe headache and changes in behavior. Since the birth of her first child, four years before, she had complained of weakness and fatigue. One year before admission she had had a "spell" lasting for about an hour, in which she appeared to be asleep and could not be roused. A second such attack, accompanied by twitching of the mouth, occurred a month later. She then began to complain of dizziness and a feeling of pressure in her head. These symptoms were attributed to emotional tension and under psychiatric treatment she improved. Five weeks before admission severe headaches and vomiting developed and a change in behavior was noted. The patient became forgetful. She would go to the store but then return because she could not remember what she wanted. One day the patient's husband found their younger child playing with razor blades while the patient, hitherto a devoted and worrisome mother, looked on with apparent unconcern. In general, the patient seemed to be easy-going and relaxed in contrast to her former compulsive behavior. In the

several days preceding admission she had become incontinent of urine. She expressed a great fear of coming to the
hospital and having an operation, which she stated would
make her "soft-brained" and put her in an "asylum."

Following craniotomy there was a complete paralysis
of the left upper extremity and a marked paresis of the
lower. She was able to feel touch, pin prick, pressure, and
vibratory stimuli in the left limbs. Two-point discrimination and position sense were impaired and she had difficulty in telling which finger of her left hand was being
held. The patient denied there was anything the matter
with her left arm or leg. When asked to raise her left arm,
she repeatedly raised her left leg. When this error was
pointed out to her, she said, "Oh, some people call it an
arm, some a leg. What's the difference!" On other occasions she would raise her right arm when asked to move
the left. When asked to distinguish between her right
arm and left leg, she could do so without difficulty. When
the examiner raised the patient's left arm and asked her
to identify it, she stated that it was *his* arm. On other
occasions the patient stated that the paralyzed left arm
belonged to the nurse. The patient also denied that an
operation had been performed. Even when she was shown
her shaven head and the operative wound in a mirror,
she still refused to admit that an operation had been performed. She would become irritable when asked about
an operation, saying, "It's ridiculous. Why, an operation
would be the last thing." She complained to her husband,
"Why are people bothering me about a non-existent operation?" She continued to be incontinent of urine but would
not deny this when questioned. On one occasion when
she was incontinent of feces, she said it must have been
done by someone else.

The patient knew the date but was consistently disoriented for the time of day. She would repeatedly ask
the nurses what time it was, usually thinking it was later
than it actually was. One afternoon during visiting hours

she asked the time and, on being told it was 3:30, exclaimed, "What are all these people doing here at three in the morning!" There were disturbances in language. The patient misnamed objects in "paraphasic" fashion. She called a thermometer a "gradient" and a wallet a "portfolio." She referred to herself as "he" or "they" and alluded to her left arm as "he." When examined on March 29, eight days after operation, she could repeat four digits forward and two backward but she could not recall the names of any of her nurses or doctors. She remembered the events of the previous day but did not recall having had a lumbar puncture. She was able to remember all the visitors she had had that day except her husband.

Patient's mood was paranoid and irascible. At times she would accuse the examiner of trying "to drive me crazy." She sardonically referred to the hospital as "Mount Cyanide." She complained that she was weak and confined to bed because she was not fed properly. On one occasion she accused the nurses of trying to poison her and stated that she was forcibly being kept in the hospital. She was especially bitter toward her husband whom she accused of trying to have her committed to a mental institution. She became concerned with sexual matters. Once she tried to fondle the nurse's breasts and accompanied this with vulgar remarks. She warned the examiner not to make any sexual advances toward her as she was "very straight-laced." She developed the transient delusion that the patient in the next bed had gone up to the operating room as a woman but had come down a man. After radiotherapy was begun on April 1, the patient charged that the treatment was giving her "cancer."

Power in the left extremities improved and on March 30, nine days after operation, the patient was able to move the fingers of her left hand. At this time she admitted that the left arm was weak and that it belonged to her but she still denied having been operated upon. However, she would talk and joke about her "bulge," referring to the decompression. The patient was discharged to another hospital for chronic care on April 25. At that time she was still disoriented for time of day. She stated that she had a "cancer" and was aware of the paralysis but still denied that she had an operation or a "tumor."

Chapter III

FORMS OF IMPLICIT DENIAL

In ORDER to determine further the relationship between the conditions of brain function and the phenomena of denial another group of 52 patients who did not deny illness verbally were studied. As indicated in Table 2, they had comparable disabilities and similar brain lesions and EEG records. When questioned, these patients did not deny their disabilities but showed other forms of adaptation to their illness. The degree to which these phenomena may be regarded as symbols of implicit denial varies of course with the particular orientation of the observer. They will be described operationally as: 1) withdrawal; 2) inattention; 3) pain asymbolia; 4) altered sexual behavior; 5) hallucinations; and 6) changes in mood. While listed separately, for purposes of record, these forms of behavior were combined to some degree in each patient.

WITHDRAWAL

This ranged from mild lethargy and lack of interest and slowness in answering questions to the picture described by Cairns, Oldfield, Pennybacker and Whitteridge (1941) as "akinetic mutism." Four such patients lay for hours at a time in the same position, often with eyes closed and failed to respond to most questions. One patient when interviewed invariably lay with his back to the examiner. A woman who appeared to be asleep when questioned by examiners would answer promptly when her sister talked to her. Another kept her eyes closed and was unresponsive to questions about illness and orientation but would an-

23

swer others readily. A patient with blindness in the right
eye kept only her right lids closed. Other patients answered questions about hospitalization and illness in
dysarthric, unintelligible fashion or only after a marked
delay while they replied clearly and promptly to others.
It was apparent that the behavior was in a considerable
degree selectively determined by the interpersonal situation. Because of the difficulty of communication few ideas
were expressed. In several, however, depressive features
were voiced. One woman, identified the hospital as a
cemetery while a man said that the patient in the next
bed was a doctor who had performed experiments in
Nazi concentration camps.

INATTENTION

This was particularly well demonstrated by patients
with hemiplegia who appeared to disregard their paralyzed limbs and the examiners' questions about them.
While lying in bed the involved extremities would fall
into awkward positions, or the patients might lie on them
without seeming aware of their existence. On being
pressed, however, the facts of the paralysis would be
admitted verbally, if only by a nod of the head. A patient
with a left sided weakness habitually neglected to wear
his left slipper. Patients with hemianopic visual field defects seemed unaware of them even after it had been
demonstrated to them many times that they were unable
to see objects and people on one side. They would neglect
food on one side of a tray or fail to identify figures on
one side of a picture. In five patients who were inattentive
to their paralyzed limbs, an apparently "hysterical" type
of sensory loss was present. The patient either seemed to
feel no stimuli on the affected side, or he perceived them
to a much lesser degree in a strict mid-line demarcation.

Six patients with hemiplegia did not look toward the

side of the paralysis even though a paralysis of conjugate gaze was not present. Some held their head and eyes averted to the opposite side. While some patients would not look to the side of the affected limbs on command, they might be able to follow the examiner's finger. Others did not look toward the paralyzed limbs either on command or in pursuit, but when the head was rotated by the examiner, the globes were observed to rotate to the opposite canthi. While this type of behavior has been explained on an anatomical-physiological basis as a supranuclear type of ocular paralysis, it is significant that it only occurred with other symbolic manifestations of denial, and cleared when they did even though the paralysis of the limbs might remain. In addition to these cases of hemiplegia, this phenomenon was demonstrated by the patient who had sustained both a head injury and the amputation of his left arm. Along with denying the amputation verbally, he kept his head and eyes turned to the opposite side during interviews.

The term "inattention" is probably a poor one as it implies only a negative quality. Actually, the selective neglect of affected parts of the body seemed to reflect a positive motivated drive to ignore the affected parts rather than simply an absence or unawareness.

PAIN ASYMBOLIA

This phenomenon was observed in eight patients along with other nonverbal forms of denial. When stimulated briskly with the point of a pin, they showed no evidence of reacting to it as a threatening stimulus either by gesture or exclamation. On questioning, however, the point might be said to be sharp and at times it was even admitted it was painful. One patient, however, not only showed no reaction, but later denied that the examiner had pricked him, confabulating that the residual mark had been caused accidentally by another doctor. These patients seemed also to withdraw from relationships with other patients and the hospital personnel. Some gave the appearance of drowsiness while others seemed merely blank, vacant and unoccupied. The man who confabulated about the "accidental" pin prick would play poker by himself all day and appeared to ignore the presence of other persons (Case 96).

ALTERATIONS IN SEXUAL BEHAVIOR

While this section is labeled in terms of its most striking manifestation, the alterations in behavior included many changes relating to attitudes about food, bowel and urinary function, and physical contacts. Whereas the patients with explicit verbal denial relied mainly on the content of their words, these patients appeared to need physical means of communication. Thirty-one patients showed changes in sexual behavior which included verbal and physical advances to members of the staff, delusions with a sexual content, confabulations about sexual activity, exposure, and open masturbation. In some cases this behavior appeared to be a means whereby the patient boasted of his virility or explained his incapacity or identified sexual symbols with health and integrity. Thus 10 patients, while admitting incapacity verbally, thought that the illness had been caused by too much, too little, or a particular kind of sexual activity. One man formerly considered a moral, religious, prudish person, following recovery from a subarachnoid hemorrhage, talked a great deal about sex and made critical or very appreciative comments about women he saw on the street. In the hospital, he repeatedly requested the nurses and female attendants to sleep with him, offering them money and remarking that if he didn't sleep with the nurses they would not care for him properly and cure him. His comment was that "women are only interested in sex and money." Other patients charged that they were being kept in the hospital for immoral sexual purposes. Some patients responded to questions about illness with sexual badinage, while answering others reasonably.

Attitudes expressed in symbols related to food included delusions about being poisoned or malnourished, excessive appetite in some and refusal to eat in others. A patient with a third ventricle tumor claimed that his illness had been caused by eating too much junk and boasted that the doctors were showing the x-rays of his stomach all over the country. Sexually he made physical advances to nurses and male orderlies and expressed the delusion that a child was being raped. The claim that illness had been caused by physical violence was common. The emphasis on physical means of expression was seen in patients who insisted on being touched, handled, or fondled in some way. Some would grasp the doctor's hand and cling to it. One man would become distressed when his surgeon on rounds would only comment on his case or address him without touching him. It was of interest that patients with hemiplegia were apt to complain of pain in the affected limbs in contrast to patients with explicit denial. Some patients were restless, childish and noisy, demanding to get out of bed or shouting for food and water. Several would call frequently for a urinal, then fill and spill it or urinate in bed. Others became preoccupied with bowel functions, stating that they would get well if only they could have a proper bowel movement. One patient claimed to be constipated and stated that only some laxative not in the hospital formulary could work. When this was finally obtained for him after much entreating, he refused to take it.

The following case report illustrates this type of occupation with genital and emunctory functions in a patient with hemiplegia:

Case 103

A 63-year-old woman was admitted to the Neurological Service of The Mount Sinai Hospital on June 28, 1950. ' For one year she had noted increasing awkwardness in her left arm and hand and one week prior to admission, a sudden loss of vision of the left side. Libido had been diminished for several months. Neurological examination showed a left homonymous hemianopia, a marked impairment of skilled and discrete movements of the left fingers and astereognosis, reduced two-point discrimination, loss of position sense and point localization in the fingers of the left hand. There was also difficulty distinguishing left and right, and dyspraxia in dressing. She showed topographical disorientation and occasionally had difficulty in finding her way about the ward. On the Wechsler-Bellevue Intelligence Scale she made an I.Q. of 100 on the verbal part but a score of only 79 on the performance scale. She seemed to ignore objects in the left half of the visual field, writing and drawing on the right side of a page. In drawing a human figure she displaced the right limbs of the figure so that they were distorted and not attached to the body. She thought the fingers of her left hand were shorter and stubbier than those of the right, even when they were placed in the right field of vision. Tachistoscopy showed that figures were not seen or not completed on short exposures. On longer exposure there was a confabulatory type of completion imitative of the figure in the right field.

Lumbar puncture yielded a clear fluid under normal pressure containing 6 wbc and 84 mgs. % total protein. The EEG record showed a considerable depression of alpha activity at the right occipital electrode and a very small amount 3-6 cps activity at the right inferior frontal, inferior parietal and ear lobe electrodes. A right carotid arteriogram showed absence of filling to the suprasylvian branches of the middle cerebral artery and was interpreted as compatible with a diagnosis of thromboangiitis obliterans of the right middle cerebral artery. Ventriculogram and pneumoencephalogram showed bilateral internal and external brain atrophy of moderate degree with the right lateral ventricle being larger. On August 15, 1950, a burrhole was made over the right parietal region and enlarged and some semi-liquid whitish tissue curetted out which on histological examination was reported as "disorganized brain tissue from the neighborhood of a massive destructive lesion."

On admission, the patient was serious, cooperative and somewhat anxious. She became visibly upset at not doing well in various tests. She tended to make excuses and would seem greatly relieved when told she had done something right. When it became apparent that her case was a puzzling one, she became depressed and talked little. She was, however, completely oriented for place, time and person, showed no misnaming or reduplication and expressed awareness of her symptoms. It was also noted that she had a poor sense of humor. Except for becoming more depressed, no other changes in behavior were noted until two days after her arteriogram, when on July 9 and 10 it was noted by the nurses that she was disoriented for time of day. On July 11 she was incontinent of urine and apparently joked about an enema she had received, referring to "Murphy-that-drip." On July 12 she expressed the delusion that the man who was visiting his mother in the next bed was a "mechanical dentist" who lived on the same street as she, the patient, did. She went into a spontaneous long rambling account of how her son had lost *his* left eye in a hunting accident, an incident which had actually happened. When tested for her knowledge of capitals she gave the capital of Denmark as "Hamlet," whereas previously she had given the correct answer. The first evidence of altered sexual behavior occurred on

July 12 when she asked the examiner, "Do you mind if I
bother you?" The reply was, "No, not at all; why do you
ask?" She then said, "Well, I like to be hot and bothered.
I'm propositioning you. I haven't been hot and bothered
in a long time." An EEG record taken on July 11 showed
a large amount of delta activity with frequencies as low as
1-2 cps chiefly at the right frontal and ear lobe electrodes,
less at the others.

During the remainder of her stay in the hospital she
showed marked alterations in sexual behavior. She made
endearing remarks and offered sexual invitations to doctors and nurses. She remarked that another patient was
noisy because "she wants to be laid." She expressed delusions about a patient in the next bed who, following a
craniotomy, was in a stuporous state for three weeks. She
said that the woman was having an affair with a doctor
and also that the woman was really a dead man. At other
times she confabulated having had an affair with a doctor
and accused the other patient of having stolen him away.
Her mood was alternately one of euphoric joking and
paranoid bitterness. Her behavior with nurses was often
spiteful and childish, especially at night. She would yell
for water and then not drink it or spill it. She would de-
mand a bed pan and then wet the bed. She would complain that the doctors passed her by and often said "All I
attract is flies." She exposed herself constantly, was incontinent of feces and because she persistently picked at
her genitals and anus, had to be restrained. She complained a great deal of constipation, frequently passed
wind audibly, and talked about the "grapefruits," "snow-
balls," and "babies" in her stomach.

She appeared to pay little attention to her left limbs,
but at no time did she verbally deny her incapacity or the
fact that they were now paralyzed or that she had had an
operation. When asked about them she would answer
with humor or sexual comments. She referred to the bandage placed around her neck after her arteriogram as her

"Robespierre" or "Sir Walter Raleigh." On occasion she called the hospital "Mt. Sinai Hellhole," "Mt. Sinai Jungle," and "Mt. Sinai Snakepit." She had non-aphasic "paraphasic" misnaming, most persistently using "paper dispenser" for waste paper basket. She called the oxygen tank in her room her "boob." Although she would usually name the hospital correctly, she displaced it nearer her home and was frequently disoriented for time of day. She apparently had hallucinations about "white cuckoos," "rats," "snakes" and "varmints" and would talk about being "gored by a rat." She mistook people on the ward for famous entertainers.

The patient was transferred to a nursing home on August 25 and the disturbed behavior cleared six weeks later. Examination on January 11, 1951, showed a complete spastic left hemiplegia, hemisensory defect and left homonymous hemianopia with complete awareness of her defects and no disturbance in orientation, language or sexual behavior. She had an amnesia for most of her stay in the hospital.

The case illustrates the change from a state of depression and anxiety to one of euphoria in which sexual symbols and humor appeared to serve as a means of resolving anxiety. The onset of altered sexual behavior was coincident with the progression of brain pathology indicated by a change in the EEG record from a focal abnormality to a more diffusely slow wave rhythm. It is also of significance that despite the presence of many disturbances in perception on the left side the patient did not express explicit verbal denial of either her hemiplegia or of the presence of the limbs.

HALLUCINATIONS

Visual and auditory hallucinations were noted in 13 patients with explicit verbal denial and in 11 instances in the other group. At times, the hallucination appeared directly related to the mechanism of denial. One patient (Case 5) verbally denied a paralysis of the right lower extremity and a paresis of the right upper limb. She told the nurse that she had lost her right leg and wondered what was going to be done about finding it. The next day she seemed agitated and said that she had seen her right leg and part of her right arm on the bedside table "just like you would put false teeth on the table." A patient who denied a left hemiplegia said that the Virgin Mary had touched her arm and said, "You'll be okay." Another patient (Case 104) with a glioma invading the thalamus had previously not denied either a left-sided weakness or having had a ventriculogram. He literally clung a great deal to the doctors and nurses and expressed himself largely in symbols relating to sex, food, and money. He would ask the nurses to kiss him, insisted on offering the doctors candy and cigarettes, and either complained or expressed great satisfaction about the food in the hospital. He boasted how expensive his wheel chair was and asked at great length about doctors' private fees. The day following an arteriogram he was told that nothing further could be done for him in the hospital and that he would be sent home. Shortly after, he expressed the delusion that someone had unscrewed the left arm of his wheel chair and had cut the left trouser leg of his pajamas. He also told a story of how he had been taken into a cellar where he had seen the cut-up bodies of other patients hanging on hooks. It was suggested that it might have been a dream related to his trip to the x-ray department. The patient, however, insisted it was true because "meat is expensive." The delusions persisted for several days after he returned home, following which he was tearful and depressed.

MOOD CHANGES

Euphoric and hypomanic, paranoid and depressed attitudes were more prominent in this group than in the patients with explicit verbal denial. Euphoric patients would evade questions about illness or answer with laughter, jokes and quips. Sometimes a euphoric reaction could be provoked by a discussion about health or by giving a test to evaluate the patient's capacities. It was often a matter of the examiner's own opinion as to whether a patient was euphoric or depressed. Similarly euphoric and paranoid attitudes appeared mingled or might succeed each other. In the course of a single day, one patient was noted as euphoric by one observer, paranoid by another and depressed by a third.

Piaget (1951) has used the term "ludic" to describe the play and imitative aspects of the behavior of young children. This is an apt way of indicating the comic, tragic or melodramatic quality that was present in many of the patients. The following case report illustrates a comic type of behavior:

Case 54

A 49-year-old salesman was admitted to The Mount Sinai Hospital on October 13, 1950, with complaints of failing eyesight and headaches of 3-4 months' duration and loss of libido and sexual impotence for one year. There was a corneal opacity in O.D. and vision was reduced to seeing fingers at two feet while vision in O.S. was 20/200. EEG record was normal and a pneumoencephalogram showed a large filling defect in the third ventricle and dilatation of the lateral ventricles, indicative of a third ventricular tumor.

The patient had a jovial, restless manner and would boast about his sexual activities and the amount of money that he had made. When questioned about his illness he admitted his failing vision and the probability that he had a brain tumor. He then would be apt to make some remark as, "I must have fallen on my head when I was a baby." When asked about his impotence he did not deny it but would add, "But if I had to I could." Another recurrent joke concerned his referring to his somewhat protuberant abdomen as a pregnancy. He would joke about being in a hotel and ask for his bill so he could go home. At times he would appear bored and talk in rather stilted and clichéd phrases. He was generally euphoric though some observers considered him to be depressed. There were some paranoid references, particularly to attendants whom he called "shit carriers." He also joked about being in the hospital so the psychiatrists could have someone to examine.

A course of radio therapy was begun on November 6 and after a week he developed evidence of further impairment of brain function. An EEG showed bilateral slow wave 4-6 cps activity. He became incontinent of urine. He was disoriented for time and on November 16 he confabulated that his brother had taken him out for an automobile ride. He showed paraphasic misnaming of objects that he had previously identified correctly, calling a thermometer a "glass tube," an emesis basin a "mouth disposer" and Scotch tape, "Scott's tissue." The confabulated journey was the prelude to a prolonged period of disorientation for and reduplication of place. While he named the hospital correctly, he located it near his place of business and stated that he had moved to the convalescent branch of Mount Sinai in Miami Beach, sometimes pronouncing it "bitch." He would say that he had been transferred to the "arthritis ward."

At this time, there were lengthy newspaper accounts of prostitution at a fashionable hotel. The patient would state that he was in the hotel; called the examiner the "credit manager" and identified the internes and residents as pimps. When asked why they wore white uniforms he replied "to protect their virginity." The patient also developed a peculiar shuffling slow-stepped gait but showed no weakness, incoordination or sensory loss on testing. His relatives remarked that he walked like his mother who had arthritis.

Observers seeing such patients for the first time often had the feeling that the patient was malingering or "acting" or "pretending." In addition to comic aspects, a number of patients had a tragic melodramatic air as, for example, they accused people of striking or starving them. The next case is an example of such a dramatic portrayal.

Case 55

A 34-year-old widow was admitted to The Mount Sinai Hospital on August 20, 1951. For six months she had complained of headache and a "different" feeling over the left side of her body. Examination showed only a diminished appreciation of all sensory modalities over the entire left side. She had a flippant, jovial, seductive manner and joked and flirted with the doctors in sexual terms. A diagnosis of conversion hysteria was made. A pneumoencephalogram, however, revealed a mass lesion displacing the lateral and third ventricles to the left and a subtemporal decompression was performed.

The patient developed a left hemiparesis but denied neither the weakness nor the fact of the operation. She complained of headache and pain in her left limbs. Her euphoria diminished and she had episodes of childish demanding behavior toward the nurses. She would either express great affection or appear very angry and once threatened to jump out of a window. She would frequently call for food or medication, then either refuse it, keep it in her mouth or regurgitate it. She talked in a slow, grim sepulchral fashion and was bitter and sarcastic. She spoke to her doctors with a disgusted expression on her face, denounced the operation and called her surgeon "Dr. Butcher." She frequently referred to herself and her head in the third person. She was disoriented for the time of day, expressed reduplication for place and had the delusion that a patient in a nearby bed, who also had brain tumor and severe headache and vomiting, was a social worker whom she had known in New Haven. After six weeks of this type of behavior, she became hypokinetic, lay as if asleep and rarely responded to questions until her death three months later.

Patients with "akinetic mutism" often seemed to "pretend" to be asleep or to portray death as they lay immobile, did not eat, did not appear to feel stimuli and expressed ideas about being buried or dead.

The ludic behavior involved not only a symbolic representation of biological functions relating to sleep and death, health and sexual activity but included "imitations" of socially integrated behavior as well. Thus one man who charged that he had been operated upon so that his surgeon could make some money would strike a boxing pose and "threaten" the interviewer. Some patients went through the motions of working. They would insist that they were going to the office to keep appointments and confabulated financial transactions. One patient following a craniotomy seemed to disregard all aspects of the operation except to go into long tirades about how much it was costing him.

These various form of behavior were noted in some degree among patients with explicit denial as well. Actually in any one case, no single mode of adaptation is used. There did seem to be, however, some reciprocal relationship among patients with explicit denial, those with marked alterations in sexual behavior and those with marked withdrawal. Thus patients with verbal anosognosia were not as a rule drowsy and in only five instances were there marked changes in sexual behavior. Patients with behavior changes relating to sex, food, and other physical modalities had usually little or no verbal denial. Withdrawn akinetic persons usually admitted illness if they could be brought to answer questions.

The chapter should indicate that verbal anosognosia is but one form of adaptation that may occur under the particular conditions of brain function that are necessary for its existence. The patient with explicit verbal denial uses words as the symbolic modality for the expression of his need to preserve his integrity. Other patients use non-verbal symbols related to health and illness, sexual activity, eating and drinking, urinating and defecating, working and making money, sleep and even death to avoid catastrophe.

Chapter IV

PATTERNS OF DISORIENTATION

Disorientation for place and time was present in each of the patients with explicit verbal denial and in many with other forms of adaptation.

While previously regarded as a manifestation of "confusion" or loss of retention, disorientation for place occurs in orderly patterns. In a study of the process of reorientation in patients recovering from brain injuries, Paterson and Zangwill (1944) noted that while the existence of patterns of disorientation depended on the presence of brain damage, the elements of the patterns were often determined by the circumstances of the environment and the patient's motivation to go home from the hospital.

DISORIENTATION FOR PLACE

When the onset of brain damage was acute as in a subarachnoid hemorrhage, the patient's responses to questions about orientation for place were multiple and mixed so that it was difficult to distinguish discrete, consistently occurring patterns. After the acute stage, however, or when the onset of disease was not as sudden, the following patterns could be distinguished.

Verbal Identification

The correct and faulty identifications were expressed side by side. Thus a patient (Case 24) stated that she was in her apartment in Ridgewood which was also "Mount Sinai Hospital." She stated, "Some call the place Mount Sinai, some call it West Chateau." Another man

(Case 14) named the hospital correctly and said it was a part of a housing project which contained both his home and the hospital.

Misnaming

These patients used euphemisms such as "rest home," "sanatorium," or "retreat," and "repair shop" when asked to name the place where they were. Names related in sound as "Mt. Morris," "Mt. Vernon," and "St. Moritz" were given. Other patients give the name of some small neighborhood hospital, often where they had been treated for a trivial illness in the past. The tendency to minimization of illness was shown strikingly by a patient who said she was in a "small private one-man hospital where they don't take serious cases." Usually the substituted name was that of an existing hospital, but at times a fictitious place was offered. A woman (Case 35) said she was in "Windham Hospital." It was learned that previously she had been admitted to Willard Parker (a hospital for contagious diseases) under suspicion of scarlet fever, and than transferred to Fordham. Apparent mispronunciations as "Mount Simonai" and "Walter Reeves" were also expressed.

Displacement

In this pattern, the patient usually named the hospital correctly but located it in another city or part of the city. The erroneous location was almost invariably close to the patient's home or place of business. One woman maintained that her home was across the street from the hospital (Case 33). An exception occurred in the case of a patient who expressed the desire to remain in the hospital because of the quarrels at home. He displaced the hospital to a point farther from his residence than it actually was. Temporal displacement was also used. One patient placed the hospital at the address of the doctor who had referred her there. Another located it in a town where he had lived 10 years previously. In another type of displacement, the patient named and located the hospital correctly but greatly reduced the distance between the hospital and his home. A woman (Case 36) after having identified her whereabouts as "Mount Morris Hospital," "Mount Sinai Hospital on F Place in the Bronx" (where she lived) finally named and located the hospital properly. However, she maintained that her home and the hospital were only four blocks apart (actually 7 miles). A man located Walter Reed Hospital accurately in Washington and gave his home as Buffalo, but insisted that they were only 7 miles apart. A woman gave the distance to her home correctly as 10 miles, but would say, "I could get there in 5 minutes."

The Confabulated Journey

This appeared frequently after the patient had apparently established complete orientation and it was also noted as the first manifestation of developing disorientation. Patients would state that they had gone home, or out for a walk, or had gone shopping. One man related how he had spent the morning "skiing with 50 beautiful girls at Mt. Holyoke College." Almost all of these confabulations involved some pleasant activity incompatible with illness.

DISORIENTATION FOR TIME

This was manifested in the form of errors in the time of day, month, and year. In disorientation for time of day, patients would confuse day and night and morning, afternoon, and evening. In a control series of patients without brain disease, patients might make mistakes of several hours but the errors never extended across a meal time. Disorientation for time of day was particularly striking after a patient had been sleeping or dozing. A boy served with his supper shortly after awakening from an afternoon nap was indignant at getting "spaghetti for breakfast." One man at 10:20 A.M. read the clock correctly but insisted it was 2:20 because "I was up all morning." A woman usually gave the time as 7:00 P.M. "because that's when my daughter comes to see me." Correct answers were most likely to be obtained during meal time. When patients were first tested, they were not permitted to look at a large wall clock. However, it was found that when temporal disorientation was present, it usually made little difference if the patient could see a clock or not. Even though he could read it correctly, he persisted in his error. It appeared that the patient used his own somatic experiences as the index of the time of day and rejected all other data which might have served to correct the error.

The following case record is an example of the relationship of denial of illness and disorientation for time of day:

Case 3

A 33-year-old German born salesman, was admitted to the hospital on January 31, 1949. For the past six months he had experienced episodes of blurring of his vision and for a year he had been sexually impotent. Examination showed a right homonymous inferior quadrant defect of the visual fields. Vision in the right eye was 20/30 and in the left eye, 20/70. Lumbar puncture yielded a clear fluid under an initial pressure of 120 mm. of water with a total protein content of 150 mg. %. EEG record was normal. Pneumoencephalogram revealed a dilated, displaced third ventricle with the appearance of a mass pushing it upward and posteriorly. A craniotomy on February 18, revealed a bluish mass 2½ cm. in diameter lying between the optic nerves. Biopsy showed a chromophobe adenoma of the pituitary.

The day after operation he seemed alert but stated that

he had not been operated upon but that an operation for brain tumor was going to be performed the next day. However, he complained to visitors that "they almost sawed off my head." When asked why there was a bandage about his head, he replied that it had been there for a week and he did not know the reason. That night he removed the bandage but denied he had done so. Except for the events of the day of operation his memory was intact. He gave the date correctly and knew the name and location of the hospital. He confabulated that he had taken a trip earlier in the day to see his banker in Lisbon. (Patient had been in Portugal before coming to the U.S. two years previously.) On February 20 he gave the date as Saturday, February 19, and again insisted that no operation had been performed, although he said he believed he had a brain tumor. He said he had put the bandage on himself to keep his hair in place. Several times he inquired in puzzled fashion, "What happened to Friday?" On the evening of February 20 he became restless and lumbar puncture yielded a blood-stained fluid under a pressure of 260 mm. of water.

On the morning of February 21 he was quite drowsy and questions had to be repeated. He stated he was in "Mount Sinai Restaurant, just eating and sleeping." He said the previous night he had gone "to see a friend in Beekman Hospital." He called the other patients "salesmen" and still denied having been operated upon. He attributed a black eye to a fight with the examiner. In the afternoon he gave the time as 10:30 A.M. but gave the correct date. He gave the day as Wednesday (actually Tuesday). He also thought he was in a German resort near Washington where he had come to go for a swim.

During the next five days the patient seemed to sleep a great deal. He would respond promptly to questions but would not open his eyes and sometimes replied in German. He identified his whereabouts as his uncle's room, the "clinic of A," " ...... Apartments," "a place where they operate on eyes," and a "radar place in Queens." The last was apparently a reference to the radiotherapy which he was told he was to receive. He identified the examiner as "Mario, someone who does eye operations around here" (Mario was a friend whom he knew in Portugal). He continued to deny, however, that he had had an operation but said that he had been upstairs to see the examiner perform an operation. He gave the date as February, 1947 and March, 1946, and when interviewed at 2:15 P.M. said it was 10 in the morning. EEG on February 26 showed diffusely abnormal 6 per second delta activity.

On February 27, the patient was more alert but was hypokinetic and offered very little spontaneous conversation. He stated he was in the Mount Sinai Hospital for "eye troubles" but denied that he had had an operation or had been sexually impotent. At 11:30 P.M. he gave the time as 3 P.M. When he was corrected, he said, "Yes, it is 11:30 but the last time you came at three." He gave the year as 1941 and said he was 33 years old and was born in 1915. He was able to subtract 15 from 41 and add 15 to 33 correctly.

The patient was given radiotherapy and his condition improved. A hemianopic visual field defect was now present. Memory tests showed only a slight impairment, the Wechsler Memory Scale yielding a Memory Quotient of 83 compared to a preoperative score of 97.

The patient retained a striking disorientation for the time of day. When interviewed in the morning, he would give the time correctly. However, when seen in the afternoon, he would give the correct hour but insist it was morning. The following interview took place at 4:30 P.M., Monday, March 7. The patient appeared to be sleeping but awakened promptly on being addressed.

(What have you been doing?)
"Sleeping." Looked at watch. "It's 4:30."
(Afternoon or morning?)
"Tuesday morning."

(But how can it be 4:30 in the morning? The sun is up.)

"In the Spring the sun comes up early."

(Would all the doctors be here so early?)

"They must have a lot of work to do so they come early."

(But isn't it unusual for doctors to make rounds at 4:30 in the morning?)

"Yes, it is unusual."

(Wouldn't all the patients be asleep so early in the morning?)

"How can we sleep if you wake us up?"

(Haven't you had breakfast and lunch already and haven't you gone to x-ray?)

"That was yesterday. I haven't eaten today yet."

(How do you know it's morning and not afternoon?)

"I've been sleeping and I can sleep only in the evening or night. I don't sleep in the afternoon."

At this point the patient's supper was brought to him.

(Isn't this a strange breakfast?)

"They give strange things to eat in the hospital."

Throughout the interview the patient's attitude seemed one of amused tolerance. The next day he recalled the conversation and admitted he might have been wrong. However, that afternoon he again insisted it was morning.

It was not until March 8, 16 days after operation, that the patient admitted having had a craniotomy. Disorientation for time of day was again present.

In disorientation for date, the patient usually gave a time in the past, often antedating the onset of illness. Thus one man who developed symptoms in June, 1947, when questioned in January of 1948, maintained it was June of 1947. It was pointed out that there was snow on the ground and that it could not be summer. The patient maintained his argument by quoting a newspaper report he had read of summer snow in New Hampshire.

It was evident that the substituted place or time often

served to express denial of illness or to symbolize some feeling about it. Thus, the patient who denied her paraparesis and tracheotomy, referred to the hospital as the "Fresh Air Roller Skating Academy." Another woman who attributed the manifestations of her brain tumor, including a subarachnoid hemorrhage, to menstrual irregularities, called the hospital "Menopause Manor." Another, following a craniotomy under local anesthesia, called the hospital "Mount Sinai Torture Chamber"; another named it "Misericordia. That's how I feel." The name given almost always retained some connection either in sound or meaning to the actual place as "Mount Sinai Restaurant" or "Mount Cyanide." A patient who admitted her illness verbally referred to the hospital as "Mount Zion," the name of the cemetery where her mother was buried. Thus the disoriented patient uses the name and location of the hospital not only to indicate where he is, but as a mode of expressing his needs and feelings.

Although all patients had brain damage, disorientation for place and time like the anosognosic delusion itself, could not be attributed to defects in memory, calculation, or perception. While patients might show deficiencies in retention, disorientation persisted after no memory defect could be found. Likewise we have studied many patients with marked memory loss who were not disoriented or who did not disclaim having had an operation. Patients who mispronounced the name of the hospital consistently might say that they or someone else had formerly been at Mount Sinai or Walter Reed. Even when patients could read the name of the hospital on charts and bed linen they still gave a false name. One such patient, when confronted with the discrepancy, remarked how "people are always stealing linen from hospitals and hotels."

Patients who otherwise could calculate well, made errors involving the year and their age (Case 3). It has been pointed out how even patients who could read the clock correctly were disoriented for the time of day. The patient who reduced the distance of 7 miles to 4 blocks from her home not only gave the addresses of her home and the hospital correctly, but could point out each location on the map. Orientation for place did not depend on topographical orientation, although disorientation for place and topographical disorientation might occur in the same person.

It was apparent that the motivation to deny illness and leave the hospital was an important factor. Like the anosognosic delusion, disorientation is a symbolic form of adaptation which the patient uses to avoid the "catastrophic reaction." The brain disease does not create even the specific symbol but rather it determines the particular pattern with which the symbol is integrated. This can be illustrated by the following case:

Case 26

A 21-year-old soldier was admitted to the Walter Reed Hospital after having sustained a traumatic amputation of the left arm and a brain injury in an automobile accident on February 22, 1953. The boy's home was in Massachusetts and he had been travelling to Washington from his station in Georgia. He denied that he had lost his arm and stated that he was in "Coolidge Memorial Hospital" in Georgia. (It was learned that this was a condensation of Cooley-Dickerson Hospital and Coolidge Memorial Bridge, places near his home). In the stages of re-orientation he successively located "Coolidge Memorial" in North Carolina, Virginia, and Washington. He then called it "Walter Reed Memorial Hospital." Like other patients, he gave up the false orientation seemingly with great reluctance, remarking "They say its Walter Reed or something" and "It's supposed to be Walter Reed." Similarly, he regretfully admitted the fact of the amputation. After orientation had returned completely and he expressed awareness of the loss of his arm, he stated that he had been told by an insurance man that a friend who had also been injured in the accident had been in "Coolidge Memorial Hospital." When this belief was given up, the patient throughout the remainder of his 5 months hospital stay, still maintained that he had a "feeling there must be a Coolidge Memorial Hospital somewhere."

Thus, the same symbolic element is integrated in various spatial and temporal patterns at changing levels of brain function, all providing a sense of familiarity and reassurance.

Chapter V

REDUPLICATION

$\mathbf{A}$MONG the other alterations in behavior shown by patients with explicit verbal denial and other forms of adaptation were the phenomena of reduplication for place, person, time and parts of the body. Reduplication for place may be defined as the confabulation of the existence of two or more places of the same name, although only one exists in reality. Reduplication for person is the confabulation that there are two or more persons although only one exists in reality. Reduplication for time is the confabulation that a present experience has also been experienced at some time in the past. Reduplication of parts of the body is the delusion that a particular member of the body is multiple, i.e., that a person has two or more left or right arms, more than two eyes, several heads, etc.

In 1903, Pick described reduplication for place and person and termed it "reduplicative paramnesia." He cited the case of a patient with senile dementia who, while in Pick's clinic in Prague, said that she had been in another clinic in another city, although the two clinics were exactly alike and a professor of the same name headed each clinic. Without referring to Pick's concept, Henry Head (1926) described a similar case. A soldier with a bullet wound in the frontal region "thought that there were two towns of Boulogne, one of which, on the homeward journey from the front, lay near Newcastle: the other one, in France, was reached after you had crossed the sea." Head stated that the man appeared to be ra-

48

tional in all other respects, except that he wrote letters to his mother while recognizing the fact that she had been dead for many years. A form of temporal reduplication can be recognized in the déjà vu phenomenon which may occur in convulsive seizures or in persons without neurological abnormality.

REDUPLICATION FOR PLACE

This phenomenon occurred in the majority of patients studied. It is stated that there are two or more hospitals bearing the same or almost identical names. While the two hospitals are in most respects given similar attributes, they differ in certain features. They may be the same in structure and have the same personnel but they are differentiated in terms of "better" or "worse," in the seriousness of the cases treated or by some event in the patient's experience. This might be an operation which is said to have occurred in the "other" institution. The "other" place is frequently described as a "branch" or "annex" of the main hospital located close to the patient's home or performing no surgery. The "extra" place thus possesses some feature which serves to "solve" the patient's problem and symbolize his feelings. Thus one patient stated that he was in a branch of Mount Sinai located in Miami where convalescent patients were sent.

REDUPLICATION FOR PERSON

This phenomenon, when it occurred, was always associated with reduplication for place. One patient claimed that his nurse had a daughter who also took care of him. He said they looked exactly alike except that the "mother" wore glasses. Another patient with one living and one dead sister confabulated that she had two living sisters. The living sister's name was Margaret, and she was also called Maggie. The patient, however, said that she had two living sisters, one named Margaret and one named Maggie. A man (Case 30) said that the patient in the bed across from him was a fellow-employee in his shop. He expressed the belief that this patient was only pretending to be ill so he could collect compensation. The patient himself was engaged in litigation claiming that his illness had been caused by a weight falling on his head.

REDUPLICATION FOR TIME

In this delusion the patient commonly confabulates that he has known the doctor or another patient previously; that he is an old friend or business acquaintance. A girl recovering from meningo-encephalitis repeatedly remarked that the examiner had been her professor at college. A soldier, awaiting an operation for an intracranial aneurysm, stated that he had been in the same hospital two years before and at that time had had the same operation performed. Temporal reduplication often persisted for weeks after all other manifestations of altered behavior had cleared. As in other instances of reduplication, disorientation and verbal denial, these ideas endured despite all efforts to point out their fallaciousness. One woman thought that the examiner had been an insurance salesman in her community and she consistently greeted him as "Mac," while seeming to accept the doctor-patient relationship in all other respects. She finally appeared to accept the explanation that the doctor only resembled "Mac" somewhat. Several weeks after her discharge from the hospital, she was visited at her home. After greeting the examiner with his correct name she chatted for a few minutes and asked "how practice was." She then remarked, "Well, Doctor, if your practice doesn't turn out you can always go back into insurance."

The following case report illustrates the role of reduplicative patterns in adaptation to illness.

Case 36

A 53-year-old widow was admitted to The Mount Sinai Hospital on March 22, 1950. There was a 3-months history of hoarseness, headache, and dizziness, and under observation the patient had become apathetic and incontinent of urine. X-ray of the chest showed an area of density in the right lower lobe, interpreted as a primary neoplasm. Neurological examination showed bilateral papilledema and awkwardness of the right upper extremity. EEG record showed symmetrical diffuse 4-6 cps delta wave activity with superimposed 2 to 3 cps bursts. Ventriculography revealed a symmetrical dilatation of the lateral ventricles. On April 13, a metastatic neoplasm 2.5 cm. in diameter was removed from the right cerebellar hemisphere. The patient was interviewed daily until her sudden death from a respiratory obstruction on May 19, 1950.

During the week following the operation the patient was restless, drowsy, and incontinent of urine. She denied that she was ill or had an operation. She was disoriented for time and place, saying that she was "home" and, later, in "Mount Morris Hospital." During the second postoperative week she seemed more alert, was cheerful, and still denied her operation. During the following week her sphincteric incontinence improved and she became oriented for time and aware of her operation. In the interview of April 28, she named and located the hospital correctly but showed reduplication for place, maintaining that there were two Mount Sinai Hospitals and that the hospital in which she was at the time was situated on F Place in the Bronx, four blocks from her home. She said that the "two hospitals" were owned by the same people and the one in which she was staying was "a sort of branch, although they don't charge you any less." She thought the present hospital was a smaller place which did not take x-rays. Characteristically, the patient was able to name the park across the street from the hospital correctly but still insisted that she was near her home. She also had the belief that the attendant had also worked as a maid in a friend's home.

The patient also expressed a reduplicative delusion for person. She was the mother of 26-year-old twins, a boy William whom she usually called Bill, and a daughter Hilda. She maintained, however, that she had twin sons, Bill and "Willie," in addition to her daughter. She described them both as having been sergeants in the Army, and that Bill had returned home on the Queen Mary, "Willie" on the Queen Elizabeth. She said that each was employed as a commercial artist (her son's occupation), and that Bill was taller, heavier, more athletic and more popular with girls but that neither was married. She said that both boys resembled her but "Willie's clothes still were at home in the closet." The patient's son had changed his surname to her disapproval. She spoke of this, remarking that "Willie" had kept his name and that "Willie" had said, "Let *him* go change his name—who cares" (a remark that the patient herself had made on the occasion). She brought out a photograph of two young children claiming that they were Bill and "Willie." When it was pointed out that one was obviously a girl, she admitted it was her daughter, commenting, "Willie must have been running around somewhere; you know how hard it is to get children in a picture."

The reduplication for person was first noted one week after operation. The patient was euphoric and voluble and her family thought she was joking. She said that she had not seen "Willie" since Christmas (when her own symptoms began) and that she understood he was recuperating from an illness. At this time, she denied her own illness and operation. This state lasted for about 10 days, following which she admitted her operation, saying, "I'm

supposed to have had one." She expressed a great deal
of concern about the absent "Willie," said he must really
be very sick and accused people of not telling her the
truth about him. On April 30, she asked, "What happened
to Willie? Where is he? They told me 6 weeks ago he was
recuperating. Something must have happened to him
Christmas week and I should know about it. He said he
would come back and he never did." During the last
three weeks of her life she appeared depressed. She never
mentioned "Willie" spontaneously and when asked about
him or her operation, she became tearful and agitated.
Reduplication for place and person persisted until the
patient's death. During this time she became more depressed and irritable and complained of increasing weakness, although EEG records showed progressively less
abnormality. On May 19 she developed difficulty in
breathing and suddenly died.

In this case the patient "used" the delusions of the
"other" son and the "other" hospital as vehicles for the
expression of her own feelings. In reduplication, the "extra" person or place or time symbolizes some motivation
or need of the patient. Thus a mediocre ex-pugilist believed that Mr. X in the bed opposite him was also Rocky
Graziano, a champion fighter. When it was pointed out
to him that Mr. X was an old man who had recently ar-
rived from Israel, he commented that he had heard that
Rocky had been traveling there. The patient, however,
did not treat Mr. X in a way different from his attitude
toward other patients and even addressed him by his
proper name. It appears as if the patient has a dual symbolic system, one portion which is used for reference
and the other to express some feeling.

REDUPLICATION OF PARTS OF THE BODY

This phenomenon was shown consistently by four pa-

tients. The following case report is an example of reduplication of a paralyzed left upper extremity:

Case 32

A 57-year-old nurse was admitted to The Mount Sinai
Hospital on April 30, 1952 with a history of anorexia,
pain in the right lower chest and weight loss of two to
three months duration. Examination revealed a slender,
poorly developed woman. Her abdomen was diffusely
tender, slightly distended, and the liver edge could be
palpated 4 cm. below the costal margin. Neurological
examination was normal. On May 7 she developed a
paralysis of her left limbs. Routine neurological examination showed a complete flaccid paralysis of the left upper
extremity and a marked paresis of the left lower limb with
slight movement at the hip and knee. A left homonymous
visual field defect could be demonstrated grossly. The
patient lay with her head and eyes deviated to the right.
There was apparent astereognosis and loss of position
sense in the fingers of the left hand. Vibratory sensation
was less well perceived in the left limbs than on the right.
Perception of touch and pin prick was retained to single
stimuli. Lumbar puncture yielded a clear fluid containing
25 crenated red blood cells and 4 white blood cells per
cu. mm. The total protein content was 20 mgs. %. The
EEG record showed a large amount of delta wave activity with frequencies as low as 1.2 cps over the right side
of the head.

The patient was interviewed daily until her death on
May 31, 1952. She expressed explicit verbal denial of
illness, stating that there was nothing wrong with her left
arm, that she could move it but that it was not as "strong,"
as "quick," or as "swift," as her right. She claimed that
she could walk but did not confabulate actually doing so.
She complained of "loss of appetite," "a run down condition," a "kink" in her neck, and worried if she were getting "rheumatism" or "polio." Throughout her illness she

kept her eyes and head deviated to the right. She could, however, turn her head and eyes to the left on command and in pursuit. This posture persisted throughout her illness, even when her bed was placed in different positions and examinations carried out from both sides of the bed. She was incontinent of urine and feces but did not deny it.

She was consistently disoriented for time of day, invariably giving an evening hour whether interviewed in the morning, afternoon, or evening. After May 22 she was disoriented for place, stating that she was in "an annex of K County Hospital, the Neurological Building" (patient had worked as a nurse in K County Hospital). She expressed temporal and personal reduplication, and stated that several of the nurses had also been supervisors at K County Hospital. She expressed the idea that the secretary who recorded the interviews was a "Miss Young" whom she had known previously, adding "they used to call me Miss Young because I looked like her." The patient showed non-aphasic misnaming (paraphasia) calling an emesis basin a "pen holder" and a roll of adhesive tape an "electric fixture," while naming correctly a group of objects not related to the hospital or illness.

The patient expressed the delusion that there was an "extra" or "false" hand lying across her abdomen while her own left arm lay at her side. She described the "extra" limb as a hand and part of an arm. At times she said she had two left hands, on other occasions she said that the hand belonged to Mrs. D., a close friend and nurse who visited her daily. Twice she said it was the hand of a doctor. The patient described the hand as "heavier," "thicker," "bigger," "fatter," and "darker" than her own. She frequently referred to it as "hot and heavy" and "a woman's hand, hard working and well used." She said that there was nothing the matter with her own left hand. When the patient was asked to demonstrate the "extra hand" she would grope about her abdomen or in space above it and say it was there or that she had pushed it away. If her own left hand was placed on her abdomen or raised in front of her, she would identify it as the "extra" one. On one occasion she called it the "sheet," another time a "pajama string." When the examiner placed his hand on her abdomen she named it correctly. When her left hand was shown to her in a mirror she pointed to the hand as one hand and to the wrist as another. There was no reduplication of any other part of the body. During the last week of her illness the delusion was less consistent with the left upper limb lying at the patient's side but it could always be produced by placing the limb across the abdomen. During this period the denial of the hemiplegia was less marked, the patient saying, "The doctors think I had a stroke."

The patient usually seemed depressed and was apt to begin an interview by crying, complaining of pain, and asking that her friend, Mrs. D. take her home. However, when speaking of the "extra" hand she would become gay and bantering. If she were unable to "find" it she might remark, "Oh, it will turn up after a while, just when you don't want it." When asked if the arm had changed at all she replied, "No, just as heavy; it's a nuisance—why don't you take it home with you? I'd like to know what your wife would say. You'd really have to make up a story." Once, in response to a query concerning her left hand, she said, "That's someone's hand, someone forgot it—that's funny, you read in the paper about people losing purses, but not a hand—it's a very heavy one—maybe it's a foot." Although she often spoke of pushing it out of the way and went through the motion several times in interviews, such actions were not observed by the nurses when she was alone. At times she would remark how "ridiculous" it was for someone to have an idea that one could have more than two hands, but she would then reaffirm her delusion. When asked whether Mrs. D. had more than two hands, she replied, "That's a silly question, how could a person have more than two hands." Occasionally, she was bitter about being sent to a "nut factory," i.e., the neurological ward, because of her hands.

On perceptual studies, the phenomena of extinction, displacement, and allesthesia could be demonstrated. She usually perceived single touch and pin prick stimuli to the left side accurately. When double simultaneous stimuli were applied to the right and left sides she only felt the stimulus on the right. Simultaneous stimuli applied to the left hand and areas elsewhere on the left side as the cheek, neck, or foot, usually resulted in extinguishing the hand stimulus. Occasionally the hand stimulus was referred to the abdomen or to the "extra" hand. This would be demonstrated with the patient's eyes closed or open. When simultaneous stimuli were applied to the right side extinction could be demonstrated less frequently. Occasionally a single stimulus to the left hand would be perceived on the right and if the left arm lying on the abdomen were stimulated the patient named her "false" arm. Allesthesia could be elicited by the use of a pin prick stimulus to the left hand followed in a fraction of a second by a stimulus to the right side. Thus, when the left hand and the right hand were pricked in this fashion, the patient frequently reported two pricks on the right hand. When stimulated in the reverse order the patient usually reported a single stimulus to the right hand. Allesthesia could be obtained only from the left hand and did not occur in the rest of the body and extremities.

AUTOPSY FINDINGS

General post mortem disclosed carcinomatous metastases to the liver and kidneys with involvement of the lymph nodes. There was severe arteriosclerosis of the aorta and slight arteriosclerosis of the coronary arteries. Examination of the brain showed the cerebral hemispheres

to be asymetrical. The right was swollen and softer.
There was a herniation of the right cingulate gyrus be-
neath the falx for a distance of approximately 1 cm. The
anterior cerebral arteries were pushed to the left by herniation of the gyri on the medial aspect of the right frontal lobe. On coronal section, the entire right cerebrum
was softened and friable. The left lateral and third ventricles were slightly dilated while the right lateral ventricle was obscured. Section of the brain stem revealed
numerous hemorrhages in the midbrain and dorsal portion of the pons. One of the hemorrhages had ruptured
through the floor of the fourth ventricle.

In this case the patient expressed denial of the paralysis
not only explicitly, but by averting her head and eyes to
the side opposite the paralysis, and by assigning the
ownership of the "extra" paralyzed hand to other people.

As in the other forms of anosognosia the reduplicated
member of the body was a part that was incapacitated in
some way though not necessarily as a result of a lesion
of the central nervous system. A patient who, following
multiple injuries in a truck accident, sustained a left
hemiplegia and fractures of the right lower limb claimed
that he had two sets of lower extremities. Another patient
had had an eye enucleated many years prior to suffering
a skull fracture. As a consequence of the brain injury he
had a right hemiplegia. He claimed that he had three
eyes, several heads and more than one pair of right limbs.
A fourth patient, following a craniotomy for a posterior
fossa tumor, developed a purulent drainage from the
operative wound. He confabulated that he had several
heads. The head that he had on he described as being
painful, having "bad drainage" and being "like a hunk
of wood, having no use, no utility." The other heads, however, were said to be free of pain and functioning well.
In the literature the cases of delusional reduplication of

parts of the body have concerned mainly patients with left hemiplegia.[*]

Reduplication always occurred in a number of forms and was never expressed in only one sphere. Thus reduplication for place was always accompanied by reduplication for time and person. The patient who stated that he had four legs also showed marked reduplication for place, time and person. He said he was in Walter Reed Hospital in Washington but stated that there was another Walter Reed in New York where he had been treated for a similar condition after the first World War. He said that his father was also a soldier. He thought that the chaplain was a clergyman from his home town, that the ward physician was a doctor he had known previously and that the ward attendant was an old schoolmate. It is thus likely that the various spatial, temporal, personal and bodily forms of reduplication are not discrete mechanisms but represent different elements of the basic reduplicative pattern.

---

[*] Bechterev (1926), Critchley (1952), Ehrenwald (1930), Meerovich (1948), Schenderov and Gamaleja (1935), and Shmarian (1934).

Chapter VI

THE LANGUAGE OF DENIAL

THE manifestations of denial were often expressed in particular forms of language. These included: (1) "paraphasic" misnaming; (2) use of the third or second person; (3) literalness and emphasis on the proper words; (4) use of slang and metaphors; (5) stereotyped, repetitive expressions, clichés and banalities; (6) stilted, ornate and pedantic usage; (7) malapropisms; (8) condensations and neologisms; and (9) humor. The classification of these patterns of language is made primarily for heuristic purposes as there was much overlapping with many responses fitting into more than one category.

PARAPHASIA

Almost all patients showed a type of language disorder in which an incorrect term was substituted for the proper name of an object. Such misnaming has been generally classed as "verbal paraphasia." In each instance, the substituted name is related to the object in terms of certain aspects of its function or structure. A radiator was called a "stove," while a slipper was called a "wallet" because, the patient explained, "they put money in it." In other cases the name given bore no logical functional relationship to the object but appeared to be related to some structural or perceptual aspect. Thus, a tongue blade was called a "ruler"; a hypodermic needle a "cigarette holder"; a wheel chair a "spinning wheel," and a pocket flashlight an "imitation cigar." Usually the substituted name represented a combination of responses to structural and func-

60

tional components. For example, a wallet was called a "bankbook"; a medicine cabinet a "bookcase"; a penknife a "nail file," and a bedpan a "saucer."

Misnaming was most frequently obtained with objects that bore a relation to the patient's personal problems, mainly those of his illness. Thus a hospital object such as the glass drinking tube was variously named a "cigarette," "stirrer," "quill," and "pipe for smoking." Doctors were typically misnamed, being referred to by such terms as "lawyer," "white-collar worker," "chief of crew," "one of the presidents," "bartender," "supervisor of insurance," and "credit manager." One of us (E.A.W.) was called by such variations as "Weinberg," "Weingarten," "Weiner" and "Wiseman," a type of misnaming that did not occur in patients without paraphasia. Sometimes the patient referred to the doctor by one aspect of his appearance, as "Dr. Eyeglasses." When patients were asked in what kind of place they were they substituted euphemisms for the hospital, such as "sanatorium," "a dump for rest and relaxation," and a "menagerie." An unmarried woman with a frontal lobe tumor who denied her illness, saying she had come to the hospital to find a husband, referred to the other women on the ward as "potential mothers."

The misnaming sometimes occurred in a humorous context, one patient calling the curtain rod by the bed a "trapeze," and another referring to the bedpan as a "piano stool." Frequently the response also served as a means of expressing and displacing feelings about himself. Thus, the nurses were called "undertakers' daughters," a syringe was termed a "used radio tube," and the side rails of the bed were designated as "my concentration camp."

When a paraphasic response was given, the patient was asked to demonstrate or state the use of the object. In most instances the function assigned was the proper one, despite the misnaming. One patient when asked to name the siderail on her bed said "I call it a bedpost but it could be called a railing." In the patients with more severe disturbances the action demonstrated was sometimes consonant with the paraphasic response. A patient who called a thermometer a "drinking tube" actually attempted to use it as a straw. Another patient called a thermometer a "nail" and went through the motions of hammering it. In several instances the disturbed perception was spontaneously shown in "bizarre" acts. A patient with a subarachnoid hemorrhage defecated into a utility hamper and argued with the nurse who tried to convince her that it was not a toilet.

The following case is illustrative:

Case 24

A 52-year-old woman was admitted to the hospital with a history of blackouts for three years and grand mal seizures for two years. A change of personality had been noted by friends for a period of three years during which she had become lazier, more dependent and demanding, banal, gossiping and repetitive. At craniotomy an olive-sized meningioma, extending bilaterally back to the optic chiasm was removed from the floor of the anterior fossa. After the operation the patient was stuporous and failed to respond to questions for two weeks. For the next two months the patient denied her illness and operation, was disoriented for time and place, was incontinent of urine and showed "paraphasic" misnaming.

She misnamed only objects related to the hospital environment. A syringe was called "part of a percolator." At different times, a wheelchair was called a "chaise lounge," a "Morris chair," and an "easy chair." A tongue blade was called an "emery board" and a "shoe horn." A pocket flashlight was called "some kind of pen or pencil." On one occasion, when the examiners were trying to convince her that she was not home but in a hospital, she was asked about the adjoining bed. She insisted that it was a "studio couch" and that visitors frequently used it. She referred to the examiner as "an agent for relief" and called the other patients "tenants."

Apart from the question of anatomical localization, there are significant points of differentiation between the observed behavior of patients with the adaptive phenomenon of "paraphasic" misnaming and that of patients with an aphasic defect. These differences are summarized in the following table.

	Aphasia	"Paraphasic" Misnaming
Type of error	Incorrect name unrelated to object, or related only in terms of sound of word	Misnaming related to some structural or functional aspect of object
Perseveration	Present	Not present
Words garbled	Present	Not present
Rhythm of speech	Altered	No change
Awareness of errors	Aware	Unaware
Correctability	Can be helped by correction	Correction usually produces no change
Anxiety in regard to misnaming	Present "catastrophic" reactions	No anxiety
Groping for words	Present	Not present
Spelling and reading	Impaired	Unimpaired
Motivational factors	Usually no relation	Selective misnaming of objects connected with illness or other areas of disturbance

USE OF THE THIRD AND SECOND PERSON

Another common pattern of language in the expression of denial was the use of the third or second person when talking about illness. The patients seemed to regard themselves or their physical defects as something outside of or apart from them. Sometimes they referred to themselves in the third person, as "he didn't have an operation," or "she feels very well today." They commonly talked about the paralyzed limb as "he," "she," or "it." Thus, a patient, asked to move her paralyzed left hand, said, "He's very limpy." Another called her arm a "dummy" and a woman said the paralyzed extremity was her "little daughter." Another patient referred to her bulging sub-temporal decompression and paralyzed arm as "monsters." Often the patient stated that the limb was not his but belonged to someone else, such as the doctor or nurse.

Frequently the illness was displaced to another person. The patient, while denying his own illness, would talk about some relative or friend being sick, often having the identical symptoms or illness that the patient actually had. A patient in whom left hemiplegia developed during an arteriographic study immediately patted her left arm, remarking to the anxious physician, "There, there, don't worry; you'll be all right." One woman, after an arteriogram, said, "My husband is so sick, how has he been feeling?" Another patient with a subarachnoid hemorrhage said that she was in "Children's Hospital" and came here because her son was in an accident. Sometimes this projection of illness was extended to a group of people with whom the patient was associated. One patient said, "My sister took this flat because the whole family got sick and she thought she'd have to run a sanatorium." Another said, "I'm completely tired; I'm not the only one; everyone in my department is tired." A woman who lived in Long Beach said that "all the Long Beach people are sick upstairs." In other cases the patient would state that other patients on the ward had the same disease or symptoms that he had. A patient with a brain tumor said that all the patients had cancer. Another refused to take medication, saying, "Why should I take these pills when he is walking

around with a headache too." When a woman with bilateral aneurysms and subarachnoid bleeding was asked
to express a wish, she said, "We should live and be well—
all of us."

Very commonly the patient, although not actually attributing his illness to others would displace his concern
to someone else. A patient who was separated from his
wife asked to be sent home because he said his wife was
lonesome and wanted him home. Another patient denied
being worried about her operation, saying, "I was just
thinking of my daughter because she's so scared." Patients
when asked about their own illness might tell the examiner how worried they were about a relative. One patient
talked about her brother, who had actually died several
years previously, whenever she was questioned about her
own operation. Occasionally, a patient would turn the
interview from questions about himself to the examiner,
asking him how *he* felt and what *he* had been doing.

Another widespread use of the third person was for
the patient to describe his illness in terms of what other
people said or did. This was especially noticeable in the
course of recovery when the explicit denial was given up.
Such expressions as "I was *told* I had an operation," or
"The doctors say I had a stroke" were used.

The following record was made of an interview with a
patient with a brain tumor and a history of convulsions
who had had a recent craniotomy.

Case 37

What is your main trouble?	From what the doctors say, I don't have the right children.
What have the doctors done for you?	So far they haven't done anything. I was really here with my married son. His wife had to get fixed up somehow and I watched the baby for him, that's all.
What have you been doing the last few days?	Nothing. Just coming to the hospital, going to my sister's, that's all.

Are you sick?	That's what they say.
Did anybody in your family have an operation?	My husband's mother did.
For what?	Something in her stomach.
What's the silk bandanna on your head for?	My son said not to show your bald head.
How did your head get bald?	It got like that from going after the baby.
What is your sickness?	My sickness is—what do they call it when other people have what I have?

On another occasion the patient said that her brother-in-law was sick in The Mount Sinai Hospital and was told he had cancer. Another time she said, "The doctors told my husband I had a sickness."

OTHER ALTERATIONS IN LANGUAGE

Some patients would talk about illness only in certain special terms and not in others. One patient, although complaining of the "hammering and sawing" that had been done on his head, still denied having had a craniotomy. Another patient denied having a tumor or an operation but charged the hospital with giving her a "cancer." Patients with hemiplegia would state that "the arm is heavy" or "lazy" or "won't move" but would not admit that it was paralyzed or weak. One patient admitted having headaches and stomach trouble but said "that isn't being sick."

There was much use of slang and metaphor. Thus, a craniotomy was referred to in such ways as "they jerked me all to pieces—they pull you apart," "they kicked out my brains," "they took a hammer and split my skull," "a cutting-up party" and "you walked on my head." In accounting for their illness patients used such clichéd expressions as "I was hit by a blunt instrument," "I feel like a punch-drunk prize fighter" or "I was hit by a Mack truck." The particular expression used was frequently of significance in relation to the patient's defects. Thus, of three patients with severe impairment of vision, one said, "I was rolled in a *blind* alley." Another referred to his wife as "my *seeing-eye* dog," and the third, when asked if there were anything wrong with his vision, said, "I've got to be straightened out, the way I *look* at it." He also denied enucleation of his left eye and referred to a Chinese patient in the next bed as a "Chinese iron-eyed bear."

Some patients used stereotyped expressions repetitively when asked about their illness. A woman when asked about her craniotomy invariably responded with "I had a benign, encapsulated, non-cancerous, totally removable lesion." In one case the patient would say, "Diabetes, colitis, arthritis and everything." Another would say, "I'll let you have it between the eyes" (incidentally, also a patient with severe visual impairment). The patient who had denied the enucleation of the eye invariably explained his behavior by saying he had been thinking of "that old expression—'I saw it with my own two good eyes.'"

The use of clichés and banalities was very common. When one patient was asked if she were sick, she said, "I'm confined to bed against my better judgment," while another answered the same question with "I'm not at liberty to divulge." A patient who was being tested for sensation to pinprick said, "I'm not numb, null and void." Patients who showed explicit denial were apt to preface their confabulations about illness with such expressions as "to tell you the truth" and "you may not believe me but."

Stilted, ornate and pedantic language was noted. One patient gave as his reason for going to a doctor, "lack of precision in dealing with my friends." Another, asked to identify the patients on the ward, said they were "patients

trying to get back to themselves from the normal standpoint of view." When asked to identify the examiner, a
patient said, "I'd say you're a doctor and in a limited sense
you're practicing medicine: you can quote me on that if
it's going to do anybody any good." Another responded to
the same question with "gathering information up to and
including inventory."

Malapropisms were frequently expressed. One patient
referred to an arteriogram as a "monograph" and a "mono-
gram." Another called an operation an "obsession." A patient who was having difficulties drawing figures said,
"You can see that drawing is not my fortitude."

Condensations and neologisms were observed in a few
cases. Thus, the hospital was called such things as a "sick-
pital," "horsepistol," a "rehabitulation center," a "neuroti-
cal hospital" and a "curable place." One patient used the
expression "a bird in the hand makes the heart grow
fonder." Another referred to treatment as "terepathy." A
girl with pronounced sexual erethism called a syringe a
"hermethisiac." Another patient, when asked where she
had been, replied, "Roaming around and then came back
to the Yampapa; we didn't splash in anyone else's terri-
tory." One patient during an interview gave as her trouble "reindeer, rainbow" and when asked where she was
said "Bucklebene." However she answered all other questions rationally indicating the selectivity of the responses.

HUMOR

Humor was expressed in patterns of disorientation, in
confabulation and paraphasia, in condensations and
neologisms and in the use of the second and third persons.
It also appeared in the over-literalness and selective misinterpretation with which some patients answered questions. Thus when asked how he had slept one man replied,
"With my eyes closed." Another answered to the question

"How do you feel" "with my hands." Also, patients told jokes or made puns which expressed their problems of illness in symbolic form. A woman with a left hemiplegia stated that she had entered the hospital "at the whim of a doctor." She referred to her paralyzed limbs as "slow on the uptake. . . . I need a new carburetor, I guess." The patient who gave her location as "Menopause Manor" remarked, "God blessed me with everything—I have piles and fibroids." A patient with central nervous system lues and weakness of a lower extremity told the following slightly expurgated joke. "A man was having intercourse with his wife in bed. Their little kid was lying across the foot of the bed. The man was yanking so hard that the kid started to fall out of bed. The man got up and caught the kid. The kid said to him, 'Pop stop yanking so hard or you'll make me a cripple'."

In addition to the content related to illness and sex, patients often used the theme of money. One man, following a craniotomy expressed no verbal denial or concern over the outcome of his illness. However, he talked at great length about how rich he was making the doctors.

DENIAL AS A FORM OF SYMBOLIC EXPRESSION

The term "symbolic" has been used in the description of the various phenomena of denial because they are the representation of a particular mode of thought and feeling. The patient admits his illness in certain words and actions but not in others. He can describe his disability in one grammatical tense or mood or person but not in another and can talk about the paralysis if he calls it by another name. The patient who complained about the "hammering and the sawing" on his head still denied that he had had a craniotomy. Patients who misname objects connected with illness usually can demonstrate their proper use. They may refer to being in a hospital in one context but deny it in another. Even though patients deny being ill in any way, they accept medication and routine and comport themselves on the ward in a manner not different from that of other ill persons. It thus cannot be said that the patient "forgets" or is "unaware" that he is ill but rather that he expresses his feelings about it in a particular language.

Chapter VII

PERSONALITY FACTORS

INASMUCH as various forms and degrees of denial may occur under similar conditions of brain function, the investigation of pre-morbid personality factors was undertaken. The main initial purpose was to compare the background of patients manifesting explicit verbal denial with those showing other forms of adaptation.

The personality histories were obtained in recorded interviews with relatives, friends and physicians after the patient had been admitted to the hospital. It was recognized that this method of study involved many factors. The informant's account of the patient was related not only to his own feelings about the patient and his illness, but to his attitudes toward the questioner and his own security and prestige needs. It was soon found, for example, that denial was by no means restricted to the patient. Relatives would state that they had noted little or no change in markedly disoriented patients. Others maintained that the patient had shown no alteration in behavior prior to being admitted to the hospital or having had some procedure as a lumbar puncture. The sister of one patient refused to believe she had a brain tumor and charged that the operation had been done merely as an experiment. Another patient, following removal of a subfrontal meningioma, said that his illness had been the result of improper care by his wife, an opinion in which his sister concurred. Denial occurred in nurses in the form of ignoring, minimizing or excusing behavior changes. Denial was also expressed by physicians who told patients with brain tumors that they had "inflammations" or "pressure." In one instance a doctor refused to admit to a patient that she had a tumor when she asked even though both knew that a craniotomy had been scheduled for the next day.

The informants were asked to describe the patient as he had known him prior to his illness and to cite the changes in behavior which had occurred since the onset. While the person was encouraged to give the story in his own way, the following check list was used for questioning:

1. Attitudes: Those toward health and illness, food, work, money and property, sex, cleanliness, neatness, punctuality, and ethical concepts such as duty, religion, honesty, and right and wrong.

2. Character of drive: Creativeness; imaginativeness; competitiveness; compulsiveness; need for superiority; prestige values; reaction to failure.

3. Reaction to stress: Temper outbursts; euphoria; humor; depression; indifference; sleepiness; worry; overt anxiety; physical symptoms; effect of alcohol.

4. Interpersonal patterns: Degree of maturity; capacity for love and interchange of feelings; dependence; passivity; self-sacrifice; domination; manipulation; stubbornness; need to be right; pedanticism; practicality; suspiciousness; jealousy; tolerance; sensitivity; adaptability; self-consciousness.

5. Expressive symbols: Sayings; superstitions; resolutions; promises; clichés; confabulations; prayers; profanity; manner of speech; gestures; mannerisms; habits.

One could not, from the informants' statements, designate or grade such qualities as "hostility" or "anxiety" or "dependence." One did learn a good deal of the way in which the patient expressed his feelings and the symbolic value he appeared to place on various acts and experiences. Even though informants, in line with their own motivations might give contradictory statements, there was a valid common background in terms of the nature of the modes of communication of attitudes within the family group.

EXPLICIT VERBAL DENIAL

The outstanding characteristic of patients in this group concerned their attitudes toward illness and the mode in which they had been expressed. All had previously shown a marked trend to deny the existence of illness. They appeared to have regarded ill health as an imperfection or weakness or disgrace. Illness seemed to have meant a loss of esteem and adequacy. A number of patients had concealed their symptoms because they had not wanted to "worry" the other members of the family. One woman with rheumatic heart disease had insisted that her husband keep her condition a secret from the neighbors. It had generally been difficult to persuade the patients to go to a doctor or stay home from work. Most often the relatives reported that the patient had never been ill or that he "never complained" or "never would go to a doctor and pamper himself," or "always made light of things." The maintenance of health seemed to be a kind of moral or ethical duty and illness represented not only unhappiness and danger but a sin. One was reminded of the situation described by Samuel Butler in his satiric "Erewhon," a mythical country where illness was a punishable crime. The use of various resolutions, homilies, clichés, justifications, and rationalizations was frequently reported. "Once you admit you're sick you are licked," "I've never had anything wrong before," "I'm sure I'll feel better tomorrow," are examples of the use of verbal symbols to solve the problems of illness. One patient developed fainting spells which she disregarded. Her family noted that her eyes were crossed but when this was brought to her attention she would usually say "you're crazy" or "there must be something the matter with your eyes." Her visual difficulties progressed and though she could no longer see television clearly and was obviously worried she would not go to a doctor. During her subsequent hospitalization she denied a left hemiplegia, right ptosis and evident diplopia. As in this case, the manifestations of sympathy or concern by others often seemed to be interpreted by the patient as a reproach or accusation. To others who were ill these patients were generally considerate and solicitous. Their advice was often considered reassuring and practical. With one exception, they were regarded by the informants as strong, "independent" people who were able to shake off or ignore their own troubles and counsel others.

Attitudes toward work were also consistent. All were characterized as conscientious and responsible people. They had a great deal of drive and compulsive energy and the majority had been regarded as successful in business or the home. Thus expressions as "always on the go," "never idle," "nothing too much for her as far as work was concerned" were noted. Most were regarded as ambitious persons with a need for improvement of themselves and others. One often gained the impression that work gave not so much a satisfaction derived from creative effort but was rather a means of attaining a position that was beyond censure. Frequently there seemed to be a feeling of guilt or uneasiness unless the patient was profitably occupied.

The need for prestige and esteem was a prominent motivation in many interpersonal situations. The word "pride" was almost invariably used by informants. Patients had tried, in the great majority of instances, to avoid becoming indebted or accepting help from others. They were people concerned with principles, duty, right and wrong, and all were described as honest and scrupulous. Attitudes toward money were significant in that they were tied up with the maintenance of integrity and esteem. In some patients saving appeared to have been a virtue in itself. Others had regarded financial success as a mark of personal worth and integrity. Most of the women were regarded as meticulous housekeepers and here cleanliness seemed of merit not so much in itself but had a moral implication, literally close to godliness.

The patients in this group were considered as conventional rather than eccentric or particularly creative or imaginative. They had generally done well in business or the professions and were respected by family, friends and employers. They seemed to have placed a value on experiences that far transcended their utilitarian material content. Thus their attitudes toward health and illness, work and leisure and other people had more to do with esteem, prestige and right and wrong than enjoyment and actual utilization of these modalities for their intrinsic qualities. It seemed important for them to regard themselves as healthy, successful and independent people.

Case 9

A 61-year-old housewife was admitted to the hospital on Nov. 11, 1948. During 1945 she had noted horizontal black stripes before her eyes and for two years preceding admission had had periods of drowsiness lasting for several minutes. For three weeks she had been incontinent of urine, forgetful and had shown peculiar behavior.

Examination showed a moderately obese, seemingly alert woman. There was bilateral optic atrophy, a dystaxic gait, and bilateral Babinski signs. She was euphoric and facetious. She was disoriented for time of day and date and gave her age as 40 years. She stated that she was in a hospital which she named only as "a first class hotel" and she identified her doctor as "an attendant who does clerical work." She denied being ill and any difficulty in gait or vision and confabulated that the reason for her hospitalization was that she was going to have a baby. On other occasions when asked why she was in the hospital, she would reply, "That's what I'd like to know. I was invited here." She also denied emphatically that she was married, but remarked that she had "two lovely daughters" (correct). She also denied having been incontinent of urine, saying that the dampness outside must have gotten into her bed. When asked about her occupation she gave it variously as "clerk," "manicurist" and "pedicurist." Although she could not recall who was president, she maintained that there was nothing wrong with her memory. Her speech contained many clichés.

Lumbar puncture yielded a clear fluid under an initial pressure of 160 mm. of water containing 85 mgs. % total protein. EEG showed a large amount of diffuse and symmetrical 3 to 6 per second delta activity with superimposed bursts particularly in the frontal regions. A craniotomy was performed on November 14 and the patient died two days later. Autopsy revealed a cholesteatoma of the third ventricle extending to infiltrate the right thalamus, basal ganglia and internal capsule.

The following account of the patient's pre-morbid personality and changed behavior during her illness was obtained from the elder of her two daughters.

The patient had been an energetic, serious, dynamic person and was regarded as the dominant member of the household. She had come to this country at the age of 12 and had worked as a "fraulein" until her marriage. Despite little formal schooling the patient had worked hard to improve herself, had taken night courses and had been active in community educational affairs. She "always kept busy." She was an excellent cook and a perfectionistic, conscientious "spotless" housekeeper. She had a great deal of "pride," was sensitive to any criticism and avoided becoming indebted to, or accepting help from anyone. The informant described how the patient would not sit down to dinner with the family, but preferred serving them and eating alone. She was stubborn and the family did what the patient considered best for them. Although her husband made a moderate living, she worried a good deal about money, was thrifty, kept the accounts and would talk about "saving for a rainy day" and "having money where you can lay your hand on it." She regretted not having gone into business and the informant thought she would have been quite successful. The patient, prior to her fatal illness, had been in excellent health with the exception of an attack of cholecystitis ten years previously. While never having any physical complaints of her own, she would be concerned if anyone else felt ill. Characteristically, however, the patient would rarely admit to being worried.

She was very solicitous about her daughters. She would say, "You girls are my whole life." She was ambitious for them to be well educated and marry well and was also quite critical of them. She would not permit her daughters to help with the shopping or housework and this was eventually felt by them as showing not only solicitude but also a certain lack of confidence. This protective attitude was also shown toward her husband, a passive person toward whom the patient was devoted but at the same time somewhat contemptuous. The younger daughter had developed considerable resentment toward her mother's domination while the elder had felt rather guilty that she had caused the patient to worry about her. Although not considered prudish, the patient seemed to avoid discussion of sexual matters. Even after her illness was said to be due to the menopause, the subject still was never discussed at home. At other times, however, she would laugh at or tell off color jokes. She seemed to have a fear that her daughters would get into "trouble" on dates, though this was not expressed directly.

The patient was well liked in her community. She listened sympathetically to the troubles of others, but never expressed any of her own. She was not openly affectionate but reserved. She had a temper but controlled it and was considered a very "practical" and conventional person. The daughters suspected that she was self-conscious about her lack of education but this was never expressed. She put considerable stress on proprieties. For instance, the family could never come to the table unless they were fully clothed. Although credited with a sense of humor, she was in no sense a "joker" or prevaricator.

In March of 1945, because of her visual symptoms, the patient consulted an ophthalmologist. He told her that she might have a brain tumor. She became indignant and refused to accept the idea. She then visited a number of physicians until she found one who attributed her symptoms to the "menopause." The family urged her to seek further medical help without success. When she developed incontinence of urine, she would go and change her clothes, but then seem to "forget" the incident. When the patient was taken for a neurological examination several days prior to her admission to the hospital, she surprised her daughters by accompanying them without protest. In the doctor's office when she was asked what the matter was, she replied, "There's nothing wrong with me; those girls think there is, so why don't you examine them."

At home, her behavior became progressively more unusual. She baked a cake with grapes on it instead of cherries and brought it to the table wrapped in wax paper. She served a meal and forgot the main course. She did not recognize her husband and wanted to know who the man in the bed next to her was. One day, she dressed herself in her own shoes and stockings and her husband's shirt. In all these situations the patient appeared calm and unruffled and showed no embarrassment. She would sit placidly idle while her daughters and husband ran the house. The family were surprised when she showed her bankbook and discussed her financial affairs with a neighbor, an act which formerly would have been impossible for her. Her whole manner became one of cheerful unconcern. On the way to the hospital she remarked that she "hoped it would be a boy."

PATIENTS WITH PARANOID TYPES OF EXPLICIT DENIAL

Some significant differences were noted between patients who expressed a complete denial in a serene, affable fashion and those who showed a predominantly paranoid form of verbal denial. Both had the same compulsive drive, the need and ability to deny imperfections, the concern with prestige; but the paranoid group had expressed their needs and feelings in a more "physical" way. They were described as having had violent tempers and having been irascible. They were more restless physically; were "always moving on to another town," "could not stay in the house, always had to be going out." Their attitude toward illness had been one of either open fearfulness or resentment. One could not go to doctors because he could not stand the sight of blood, a second because of fear of needles. Another had always expressed a hatred of doctors. Another patient had formerly been hospitalized for an operation on a pilonidal cyst but fled before it could be performed. The use of "physical" symbols was also seen in the greater interest in personal appearance, bodily cleanliness and odors, bowel habits, and fussiness about food and diets shown by these predominantly paranoid patients. There was great concern with the overt attributes of masculinity and femininity. The patient described in Case 30 was unhappy over his small stature and was ready to fight over any affront. He

also worried about his bad teeth but wouldn't go to a
dentist. A favorite expression was, "If I were taller and
had good teeth, I'd own the world." He had had an unhappy marriage which he had attributed to his inability to
satisfy his wife sexually. It was probably of interest that
his subarachnoid hemorrhage occurred on the morning
after his second marriage. Although "frightened to death"
of hospitals and operations he would attend autopsies
and had served as a volunteer ambulance driver during
the war. Another patient would assert his authority in the
family by whipping his son. The patients with paranoid
forms of verbal denial had shown much more overt sexual
behavior, four of the seven having engaged in extramarital
affairs. The patients with complete explicit verbal denial,
on the other hand, were described usually as having been
quite proper in the conventional sense.

Some interesting variants were shown by patients who
expressed denial through reduplication of parts of the
body. The man (Case 39) who stated that he had four
eyes, arms and legs had been an engineer with a great
drive for physical perfection. His interests included Judo,
body posture, Buddhism, longevity, guns and cameras.
Having lost an eye in an accident he was extremely self-
conscious and would always confront people full-face so
that the prosthesis would not be noticed. He was described as a great bargain hunter and would buy two of
everything so that he would have a spare in case anything
happened to the first. The nurse (Case 36) who claimed
that she had two left arms, though conscientious in her
work, seemed to have lacked the drive and "independ-
ence" that characterized most patients with explicit denial. She had been greatly attached to a friend, a motherly
type who for years had advised her and coped with her
problems. The delusion that the paralyzed "extra" hand

belonged to her friend seemed to symbolize the relationship between the two women.

PATIENTS WITH OTHER FORMS OF DENIAL

This group of patients who did not explicitly deny illness also contained many persons with prestige and security needs. The combination, however, of denial of illness as a symbol of personal integrity and the ability to formulate denial in verbal fashion did not occur. Illness was more often regarded as a problem in itself, not as a disgrace or an inadequacy. Some patients seemed to have been fearful or ashamed of previous ailments and were apt to become anxious, depressed and withdrawn when ill but they did not tend to deny or rationalize it. Most of them had gone to doctors willingly. A number appeared to have used the circumstances of illness as a means of communication with others. Thus five patients were described as being hypochondriacal and complaining, one man having been hospitalized on eight occasions for vague complaints prior to sustaining a hemiplegia.

These patients were described in general as being more "emotional" and open in the expression of their needs and feelings. Nineteen were characterized as being "dependent" or childish. This does not mean that these patients were necessarily more "dependent" in an absolute sense but it indicates, rather, that their means of expression of their needs had been more overt, so as to be recognized by relatives. Twenty were regarded as hard and conscientious workers but the competitive aspects seemed to be less prominent. In general there was less of the "ascetic spirit" and more capacity to enjoy things for their intrinsic qualities. Habits of cleanliness and meticulousness and attitudes toward money and property did not differ significantly in the two groups. While pa-

tients with explicit verbal denial were usually regarded
as efficient and successful, there were more imaginative
and creative persons in the other group.

It is of course impossible to assign a set of pre-morbid
personality characteristics to patients with each of the
manifold types of denial. When, however, one form of
adaptation was predominant, there was evidence that this
type of expression had been a significant one in the maintenance of adjustment before the illness. This relationship
was well shown in the histories of patients with aberra-
tions in sexual behavior.

PATIENTS WITH ALTERED SEXUAL BEHAVIOR

The background of patients with marked alterations in
sexual behavior was characterized by the importance
placed on sexual attitudes in interpersonal relationships.
Thus sexual attractiveness, prudishness, flirtatiousness and
hypersensitivity to sexual implications had been significant components in the maintaining of esteem. In some
the ability to make sexual conquest was equated with
prestige and success. A number of women had expressed
their dissatisfaction about marriage by openly resenting
sexual attentions. Several, while in the hospital, attributed
their illness to sexual activities or to their absence. The
patient (Case 103) whose exhibitionistic and coquettish
behavior was cited as an example of an implicit form of
denial was described as having previously been a viva-
cious, temperamental, flirtatious person. She was a former
actress with many admirers. Outside of men and clothes
she was not competitive, had never shown any tendency
to deny illness and was quite willing to let others take
care of her. In some cases sexual symbols had served as
a means of relief in situations of stress. The wife of one
patient was describing their grief after the death of their
son from poliomyelitis: "We sat around and told dirty

jokes—we thought it was terrible—but it was the only way we could escape." It was apparent that sexual attitudes had played important roles in the maintenance of adjustment.

Apparent reversals of sexual attitudes were also common. Patients hitherto considered as modest and prudish became vulgar and amorous when changes in brain function developed; but what was common to both types of behavior was the high valence placed on sexually symbolic attitudes. On entering the hospital, one woman was so modest that she refused to use a bed pan in the presence of a nurse. She expressed great disgust at the off-color jokes told by the other woman in her room. Following a craniotomy she repeated the same jokes to doctors with seeming zest and added others of the bathroom variety.

Another woman was described by her daughter as having been so prudish that she wouldn't appear in a bathing suit unless it had a long skirt. After a subarachnoid hemorrhage she exposed her body, told lewd jokes and clutched amorously at the doctors. A butcher had had the reputation of being extremely courteous and decorous with his customers. At home he was exceedingly modest about exposure in any state of undress. Following a craniotomy for a sub-frontal meningioma he made sexual advances to the nurses and became abusive when these were declined.

The pre-morbid background of patients with other forms of adaptation, notably those with drowsiness, pain asymbolia, marked euphoria and depression and those with changes in eating habits, is being studied. There is considerable evidence that these phenomena like verbal anosognosia and alterations in sexual behavior are not only physiologically determined but are to a great extent influenced by pre-existing social and cultural factors.

The patients with explicit verbal denial seemed to form the most homogeneous group both in clinical behavior and in regard to personality background. This may be so because informants were often able to quote their words while the non-verbal manifestations of attitudes are not so readily interpreted. In the later stages of the study it has been possible to predict, on the basis of the personality interview, whether or not a patient will develop explicit verbal denial if the sufficient conditions of brain function develop. Further study of these factors among patients with implicit denial is necessary but the work to date indicates that there is a significant relationship between previous behavior and all types of denial expressed after brain damage.

Chapter VIII

ANATOMICAL AND PHYSIOLOGICAL FACTORS

THE conditions of brain function associated with the described phenomena were provided by lesions of varied etiology. Of the 52 patients who expressed explicit denial, 36 had brain tumors; nine had disease of cerebral vessels, seven with subarachnoid bleeding; five had had lacerating brain injuries; one had had meningo-encephalitis while in one the clinical diagnosis was unclear. The cases reported in the literature are chiefly those of vascular disease and tumors, but that the etiology may be diverse is indicated by descriptions of anosognosia in metabolic disorders as Paget's disease (Bender, 1934) in the encephalopathy associated with severe burns (Hamburg, Hamburg, and DiGoza, 1953) and in patients with chronic barbiturate intoxication (Wikler, 1953). Statistics on the incidence have been supplied by Nathanson, Bergman and Gordon (1952) who found verbal anosognosia for the paralysis in 28 of 100 patients with hemiplegia admitted consecutively to a general hospital.

Analysis of the anatomical and pathological data showed certain features. The pathology was usually of rapid onset as indicated by the high incidence of rapidly growing neoplasms, ruptured aneurysms and acute head injuries. The syndrome of verbal denial was not observed in patients with cerebral arteriosclerosis, in those with slowly developing degenerative or demyelinating diseases nor in those with congenital defects as an infantile hemiplegia. In 11 cases anosognosia was first noted following

85

a craniotomy and in one patient it appeared after a grand
mal convulsion. Among the neoplasms ten were of the
malignant gliogenous infiltrating type involving frontal,
parietal and temporal regions, six were of metastatic ori-
gin and two were sarcomatous.

A milieu of function sufficient for the development of
anosognosia could be produced by a lesion anywhere in
the brain if it were associated with increased intracranial
pressure or subarachnoid bleeding. Thus the series included three patients with acoustic neurinomas and
papilledema and one with a lesion of the medulla associated with intracranial hypertension. All of the cases of
brain injury and most of those with disease of intracranial
blood vessels had had bloody or xanthochromic spinal
fluid.

In the absence of subarachnoid bleeding and intracranial hypertension, the conditions for the existence of
anosognosia were particularly well provided by lesions in
the region of the third and lateral ventricles, the diencephalon and midbrain. Thus tumors of the third ventricle
of comparatively small size, slow development and benign
histological characteristics were present in eight instances.
Pituitary adenomas and subfrontal meningiomas com-
pressing the optic chiasm may likewise furnish the requisite physiological background. These patients and those
with aneurysms of the Circle of Willis are especially
suited for study because they do not have the gross defects in perception and referential symbolization found
in patients with extensive cortical damage.

It did not matter which cortical area was involved by
a tumor provided that there was accompanying involvement of deeper structures. Thus anosognosia occurred
with frontal, parietal or temporal lobe lesions when these
invaded the medullary center of the cerebral hemisphere
and the corpus striatum and diencephalon. The cortical
location was significant in determining the particular type

of disability that the patient might deny. Circumscribed benign tumors or cysts situated close to the convex surface of a cerebral hemisphere that could be demarcated were not associated with anosognosia except briefly during the aura of or following a convulsion. In one patient denial was not expressed even after the removal of the left cerebral hemisphere. It can be said that meningiomas of the convexity are not associated with any of the forms of anosognosia described in the absence of ventricular distortion and increased intracranial pressure.

ELECTROENCEPHALOGRAPHIC STUDIES

The electroencephalographic record provided significant data as to the nature of the physiological milieu. In all but one patient in whom records were obtained, diffuse, usually bilateral, slow-wave activity ranging from 1 to 7 cycles per second was present. In no instance was enduring anosognosia of the types described associated with only a focal slow wave abnormality. In several patients no evidence of denial, reduplication or disorientation was present on admission to the hospital. The EEG record in these cases was read as showing a focal abnormality. When anosognosia developed, the EEG was repeated and bilateral slow wave activity was demonstrable. Conversely in Case 2 denial of illness and disorientation for place were present on admission with a bilaterally slow wave EEG rhythm. After the drainage of purulent fluid from the region of a tumor, the abnormal waves were localized to the site of the lesion and the denial and disorientation were no longer present. In summary, the conditions of brain pathology were those which by virtue of rapidity of development, diffuseness, bilaterality or midline situation or through the effects of increased intracranial pressure or subarachnoid bleeding produced diffuse delta wave activity in the EEG record.

From the standpoint of anatomical and physiological

localization the pathology appeared to relate to a disruption of the centrencephalic system (Penfield) involving the reticular formation, thalamic nuclei and thalamocortical connections. In contrast to the classically described long-fiber discrete sensory systems, the centrencephalic system conducts through short neuron chains and has widespread cortical effects. These features are related to our observation that lesions involving different portions of the system may be associated with the same pattern of alteration in symbolic behavior. Thus the patterns of explicit verbal denial, disorientation and mood change with a frontal lobe tumor may be identical with that accompanying a mid-brain lesion.

DENIAL IN OTHER STATES OF BRAIN FUNCTION

It should be pointed out that these observations do not mean that all manifestations of denial of illness are associated with these particular conditions of brain function, nor is this state of brain function necessarily associated with denial. They indicate only that this pathological state existed in the 52 patients with explicit denial of disabilities of the type and duration that have been described with these particular methods of study. In many other patients with hemiplegia denial appears in transient fashion. Often such patients seem to prefer to use only the good arm. Patients with hemianopia commonly ignore objects and persons on the side of the loss of vision. Under hospital conditions, however, these patients do not persist after repeated experience in maintaining that there is nothing wrong with their vision unless there is a more generalized disturbance of function. Many aspects of illness are denied or "forgotten" by normal persons under certain conditions. In combat a soldier may ignore a wound or the pain of an injury. Another interesting example is the phenomenon of phantom limb where the person has the "feeling" that his limb is still present. Thus Captain Ahab would feel his missing leg when his wrathful thoughts turned to the White Whale who had shorn him. However, under ordinary environmental conditions the delusion that an amputated extremity is whole occurs only with such pathology as has been indicated. Certain features of the syndrome of denial may persist in delusional fashion after such alterations in brain function are no longer present. The prolonged duration of reduplication has been mentioned and in two patients with head injuries, confabulations about the nature of the accident were expressed for several months after the EEG record no longer showed diffuse slow wave activity (Cases 29, 52).

ONSET OF DENIAL WITH PROGRESSIVE BRAIN DAMAGE

As a progressive lesion produces greater and greater changes in brain function, the onset of anosognosia may appear with dramatic rapidity and intensity. Patients who were depressed and fearful about their illness became affable, unworried, expressing a flat denial of the very symptoms which had hitherto concerned them. The following case report illustrates such a development:

Case 6

A 28-year-old housewife was admitted to The Mount Sinai Hospital on September 8, 1937. For six months she had eaten poorly, complained of nausea and had become anxious and irritable. For a month she had vomited, walked unsteadily and complained of headache and blurred vision. Examination showed signs of a brain stem lesion including paralysis of ocular gaze to the left, nystagmus and ataxia of the right limbs. She was completely oriented and aware of her disabilities. She was depressed, despaired of ever recovering and spoke of suicide. After a course of radio-therapy she was discharged on November 3.

The patient was readmitted on November 19 because her neurological signs had progressed. She now had papilledema and rigidity in all four limbs. She appeared apathetic and although she knew she was in a hospital, did not think that she had left it. After a week she became garrulous and euphoric although she usually slept when not engaged in conversation. She denied being ill or having anything at all the matter with her. She was incontinent of urine and feces but when questioned would say that someone else had soiled her bed. She was disoriented for place and time and misnamed objects (paraphasia). While usually cheerful and affable, there were paranoid episodes in which she would accuse the staff and her family of neglecting her. On several occasions she berated her husband for spending all his time in the "ladies room." She became more drowsy and died on February 14, 1938.

Post mortem examination of the brain showed flattening of the convolutions and a medullary pressure cone. There was a marked internal hydrocephalus of the lateral ventricles, distorting them asymmetrically. The third ventricle was almost obliterated and pushed to the left and the aqueduct of Sylvius was slightly displaced. The tumor was infiltrating without a clear demarcation from the rest of the brain. It extended from the optic chiasm to the level of the posterior commissure, destroying the hypothalamus and invading the thalamus, particularly the medial nuclei. The entire right thalamus was swollen. There was a cystic area 1.0 by 0.5 cm. in the interpeduncular space between the mammillary bodies and the infundibulum.

EFFECTS OF RESTITUTION OF BRAIN FUNCTION

In recovery of brain function, particularly when it is rapid as after subarachnoid hemorrhages, in encephalitis or following the removal of a tumor there is a common sequence of behavioral stages. During the period of greatest brain damage the patient may deny illness in verbal or non-verbal symbols. As function improves, as indicated by the changes in the EEG record, in the spinal fluid and the neurological signs, he then may become agitated, depressed or hypochondriacal. Thus in paradoxical fashion the patient becomes anxious and disturbed at the very time that his disability may be clearing.

This type of behavior was illustrated by the soldier who said he was in "Coolidge Memorial Hospital." The patient first admitted the loss of his arm one month after the injury. Prior to this he had had an air of brash bravado. He then appeared depressed, tearful, and agitated and expressed concern about his parents' health (although they were quite well). He ruminated about going insane and getting a dishonorable discharge from the Army. He talked obsessively about his teeth and asked many times if the operation (jaw wiring) should have been done. He complained about blurring of vision, although no basis for this could be found, and gave this as a reason for not reading or writing letters.

An analogy can be drawn between this type of behavior and the "abstinence" syndrome that appears in addicts abruptly deprived of drugs, particularly the phenomena associated with chronic barbiturate intoxication. It has been noted by Isbell *et al.* that patients with barbiturate intoxication may become euphoric or paranoid and deny the existence of such symptoms as dysarthria, ataxia and urinary incontinence. Soon after the drug administration is terminated an acute hallucinatory delirium, often with convulsions, may appear. It is likely that this reaction does not represent a specific toxic effect but is rather the manifestation of a more general principle of brain function which operates not only when the level of activity is suddenly altered by the cessation of the maintaining chemical agents, but by the rapid healing or removal of any pathological process.

Although the "abstinence" syndrome is particularly apt to develop when recovery is rapid, as after a subarachnoid hemorrhage, it should be noted that the period of restitution of brain function is not automatically accompanied by such behavior. Patients who maintain the more complete and enduring forms of verbal denial and disorientation are less likely to become disturbed than those in whom denial is less complete and more transitory. The environmental circumstances are important. For example with improvement in brain function, patients are frequently taken off the critical list, special nurses are dismissed, visitors are restricted, the staff becomes less interested and the patient often goes home to encounter additional problems.

Convulsions occurred in four patients during this period following the clearing of the anosognosia. One woman who had had a subarachnoid hemorrhage returned home to learn that her landlady had let her room and that her job had been changed to a less desirable one. She had a grand mal convulsion. Another patient with a residual right hemiparesis went to live with his mother because his wife felt she could not care for him and their two children. On his first visit to his own home he had a grand mal convulsion. At the level of function in which anosognosia was present, convulsions occurred in only one patient (Case 44). Prior to the development of disorientation and other delusional forms of denial, however, convulsions were frequent. One patient had repeated petit mal seizures during her first few days in the hospital. During this period, she was completely oriented and aware of her illness. When she became consistently disoriented, the seizures ceased. Another patient with a temporal lobe tumor had déjà vu seizures until he developed increased intracranial pressure and became drowsy. The convulsions in these patients may be regarded as a homeostatic attempt to restore a milieu of function in which the symbols of denial may again operate.

The appearance of agitated behavior and convulsive manifestations following the clearing of anosognosia is illustrated in the following case of a mixed type of denial.

Case 30

A 46-year-old mechanic was admitted to The Mount Sinai Hospital on July 1, 1950. On the morning after his wedding he had complained of a sudden right-sided headache during coitus after which marked weakness of his left limbs developed. Ten days previously he had been struck on the head by a falling weight. He was seen by four doctors before he consented to be taken to a hospital near his home where lumbar puncture yielded bloody spinal fluid. After four days he had persuaded his wife to take him home.

Neurological examination showed paralysis of the upper left extremity and pronounced weakness of the left lower extremity. There were marked diminution of all sensory modalities over the left side and a left homonymous hemianopia. The deep reflexes were more active on the left, with a Babinski sign on that side. Lumbar puncture yielded xanthochromic fluid under normal pressure. The electroencephalogram showed diffuse slow waves of frequencies as low as 1.8 cps with focal accentuation in the right frontal region.

On the day of admission, the patient denied completely that there was anything wrong with his arms or legs. On the following day, when asked whether he could move his left arm, he said: "It doesn't function as I want it to, but there isn't anything wrong with it. If I could only go to the bathroom, I'd be all right." Two days later, when asked how his arm was, he replied: "Better." When asked then what was wrong with it, he said: "Nothing, it's just heavy." On July 17, seven days after admission, he remarked: "My left hand doesn't do what I want it to do, but there is nothing wrong with it." When asked why he came to the hospital, he answered: "For a rest, but I might have a blood clot on my brain." When asked whether he was worried about his condition, he replied: "No, it never happened to me before; so why should I worry now."

He had been incontinent of urine but denied it. The following day he admitted that his left extremities were a "little weak," but he thought that he could walk well. He remarked that his left arm and leg had previously been weak. He noticed only people on the right side of his bed, read only the last letters of words and the right half of a clock but insisted there was nothing wrong with his vision. He complained frequently of headache and constipation. He said that the headaches had come because the doctors had pounded his head. He blamed his condition on ill treatment received in the other hospital. He complained that another patient had stolen his toilet paper. He accused his wife of going out with one of the "good-looking doctors" and wanted her to remain with him all the time. He thought that a patient in a nearby bed had called him a "queer." Food collected in the left side of his mouth and he would lie on his left arm.

He was disoriented for place, naming the hospital correctly but displacing it to an address one block from his home. He was incontinent of urine, sometimes admitting and sometimes denying the condition. He confabulated that during the war he had served in the infantry in France. He stated that he and his wife were each 36 years old, whereas he was actually 46 and his wife 31. He misidentified other patients, claiming that one was a prominent cafe-society figure and said that he had been visited by a movie star. He confabulated that both his parents were living.

On July 27, on the 14th day after admission, he admitted completely the weakness of his left limbs and the visual defect a day later. At this time he was fully oriented for time and place. Despite the return on the same day of ability to move his left hand and fingers, he was very anxious. He would avoid answering questions about his condition. The only abnormality expressed was a reduplicative delusion in that he thought that the patient in the next bed was a man who worked in his shop. He believed that this man was pretending to be ill so that he could collect compensation. The patient became so anxious and frightened that he left the hospital against advice, only to appear in the private office of one of us the next day in a state of great agitation.

Throughout the next three months the patient was described by his wife as exceedingly irritable and sensitive to noise. He drank a good deal of alcohol. He attempted unsuccessfully to return to his work. He then appeared less anxious and he began to experience déjà vu phenomena as "I see someone on the street and I feel that I know him, but I just can't place him. I get all steamed up, dizzy, and nauseous like I'm closing up in my chest and I get a pounding in my head—then I have to go in a different direction because if I stay, I'll pass out." These spells occurred two or three times a week and the patient reported actual fainting on several occasions. He also had episodes when he felt forced to count or repeat and spell out words he had heard or seen. Examination showed a persisting left homonymous hemianopia of which the patient was now aware. His wife reported that he was apt to leave food on a plate to the left of him. He also had had the experience of mistaking the sign WOMEN for MEN with embarrassing results, and on another occasion had suggested buying a $136 TV set for the $36 which he thought he had read. An EEG record obtained on April 22, 1952 revealed only a focal slowing over the right temporal area with occasional slow activity of the other right sided electrodes.

The déjà vu experiences lasted for about 18 months. When interviewed at that time, the patient remarked "I miss those spells. They made me feel so good." At this time he began to dream almost every night. Most of them had themes of violence and he related one recurrent dream. "I dreamed about a good friend of the family. I said you're a wise guy making a play for my wife. I shot him, killing him and I remember him lying there with blood on his head." In this dream, the patient, in symbols related to sex and violence, represents the events of his illness in a way comparable to that shown in the delusional state.

RELATION TO DREAMING

Although after recovery, patients were apt to refer to their experience as a "dream," dreams were very rarely reported during the period in which the anosognosic delusions were expressed. After restitution of brain function, the patients described dreams in which denial was expressed in patterns of confabulation, disorientation and reduplication. Thus, the soldier who had lost his left arm had a dream in which the same car in which the accident had occurred was dragged by a train but no one was hurt and he saw himself with his limbs whole. A woman who had previously denied her operation after returning home had a dream in which a friend came home well after an operation. It is likely that one of the attributes of normal brain function is the ability to distinguish a dream as such.

RELATIONSHIP OF ANATOMICAL AND PHYSIOLOGICAL FACTORS TO THE SYNDROMES OF DENIAL

The observations indicate that brain damage is not the "cause" of denial per se but rather the level of brain function determines the integration of the pattern in which denial is expressed. Thus, patients with explicit

verbal denial had tended to ignore and rationalize illness and deny felt inadequacies and imperfections long
before brain disease developed. The effect of the brain
lesion is to provide a milieu of function in which *any* incapacity or defect *may* be denied whether it is a hemiplegia, the fact of an operation or an unfortunate life situation. The particular elements of denial that are used are
related to the person's previous experience—the symbolic
modalities in which he habitually expressed his motivations. Thus one patient with a tumor of the third ventricle
and a slow wave EEG rhythm may express a complete
denial of illness while another under identical conditions
of brain function may admit all of his defects.

The "Body Scheme"

The usual explanation of anosognosia in the literature
is that it is the manifestation of a disturbance in the "body
scheme." The validity of this view depends, of course, on
what one's concept of body scheme is. In general it has
been regarded as a three-dimensional image of the body
represented in the parietal lobe or its connections, much
as there is motor and sensory representation on either
side of the Rolandic fissure. A lesion in this area is said to
disrupt the "body image" so that the person becomes unaware of a particular part of his body or of its disability.
This formulation has been used especially to explain denial of hemiplegia and blindness. Because it has been so
widely accepted, it may be important to consider in some
detail why it is not adequate.

No matter where the "body image" may be located,
patients with similarly situated lesions may show clinically different forms of adaptation. Thus one patient denies a hemiplegia while another with a comparable lesion
and an identical EEG record recognizes both the existence of the limbs and their paralysis. Also as exemplified

in Case 51, many perceptual disturbances may be found in testing the affected side without the expression of verbal denial by the patient.

Anosognosia for hemiplegia has been considered as a focal sign of involvement of the parietal lobe (Critchley 1953), (Roth 1949), (Cobb 1947). Many patients, however, with lesions of the parietal area do not show anosognosia in any of the forms described. Even after extensive cortical ablations, they do not deny the weakness and sensory loss in the contralateral limbs. In no recorded case does anosognosia occur with only a focal lesion such as a cyst or benign tumor limited to the parietal area. Critchley (1953) cites a case of Halloran's (1946) as an example of anosognosia for hemiplegia allegedly resulting from a cortical lesion. The patient had a right hemiplegia and claimed that the right arm belonged to the doctor. Autopsy however showed a large subdural hematoma which involved not only the parietal lobe but severely compressed both cerebral hemispheres and displaced the ventricular system. Also anosognosia with hemiplegia may occur with lesions that do not directly involve the parietal lobe such as a basilar artery occlusion. It is true, as Critchley states, that the great majority of cases with anosognosia for hemiplegia have involvement of the parietal lobe. It is likely that this is so because parietal lobe lesions are particularly apt to be associated with a useless hand. However, anosognosia in enduring form occurs with a single lesion only if, in addition, the necessary milieu of brain function is created either by extension to or compression of deeper structures.

Another flaw in the body scheme hypothesis is that the portions of the body for which there is denial or unawareness are invariably disabled in some fashion. For example, the patient described by Cobb as having an "amnesia" for the left limbs had an astereognosis of the hand and a marked loss of position sense in the toes. Of course, whether or not one finds a deficit in the affected limbs may depend on the method of examination that is used. Thus routine neurological sensory examination may be negative but if stimuli are applied bilaterally and simultaneously, a sensory or visual field defect may be demonstrable. If the body scheme theory of anosognosia, as stated, were valid, then one would expect to find some patients who would be unaware of or deny the presence of normally functioning parts of the body. Further the disability that is denied is not necessarily caused by a lesion in the central nervous system. Thus one patient denied the loss of an amputated arm while another claimed that a previously enucleated eye was still present. It would be an incredible coincidence if a lesion should destroy only the areas in which awareness of these members were represented.

The denial of multiple disabilities by the same patient often successively, and the denial not only of physical defects but also of operation, incontinence of urine and feces, and unhappy life situations likewise are not explicable by such a concept of body scheme. There obviously are not multiple lesions which successively and selectively destroy centers in which are represented awareness of various parts of the body, ailments, inadequacies and traumatic experiences.

If the same lesion causes both the defect and the denial or reduplication, then it should be expected that one would not outlast the other. However, the disability frequently remains while the denial disappears. In such patients the anosognosic delusion may be once again produced by the intravenous administration of amytal sodium. It is hardly likely that this effect of barbiturates is produced by a specific action on the parietal lobe.

In none of our patients did anosognosia appear as an

isolated manifestation but was always accompanied by other alterations in behavior such as disorientation, reduplication and paraphasia. If the body scheme hypothesis were true we would have expected to find some cases in which anosognosia appeared alone. Such patients have occasionally been reported in the literature. It should be pointed out, however, that disoriented patients often appear alert and patterns of reduplication and displacement or a confabulated journey may be elicited only on systematic questioning. Pick in describing patients with reduplication remarked that "such patients by dignified demeanor and a certain wit are apt to deceive one as to . . . mental defects." There is also the factor of what the examiner considers to be a change in behavior. For example Babinski (1924) stated that a patient with anosognosia for left hemiplegia had no other mental disturbance. Yet he described her as "showing exaggerated loquacity, reduced capacity for attention and sexual behavior quite out of character, astonishing the people around her."

If a concept of body scheme is used, it cannot be "localized" to any part of the brain as an anatomical representation. It must include not only the physical appearance of the body but also other spatial, temporal, and interpersonal aspects of the relation of the self in the environment. Further it must include the role of the motivation of the individual to preserve his integrity. Otherwise, significant patterns of human behavior are relegated to the status of neurological curiosa.

Chapter IX

PSYCHOLOGICAL STUDIES

ALTHOUGH many statements have been made in the literature on the mental status of patients with denial of illness, there have been few cases where actual formal psychological investigation was carried out. In the present study various tests were administered during the period when altered behavior was evident clinically. These consisted mainly of standardized procedures such as the Wechsler-Bellevue Intelligence Scale, Rorschach, House-Tree-Person drawings, Bender Visual Motor Gestalt test and the Wechsler Memory Scale. In addition, some patients were examined for recall of stories and interpretation of proverbs.

In their attitude during the testing situation, these patients did not show the "catastrophic reaction" which so commonly occurs in patients with brain disease who are aphasic or have other defects. There was a bland serenity in the patients with verbal denial, and paranoid, euphoric or withdrawal attitudes in the patients with other forms of adaptation.

The level of intellectual functioning, according to the Wechsler-Bellevue IQ's, varied from scores as low as 66 to as high as 125, averaging in the 90's. For the most part the score corresponded to the level expected from the patients' educational background. In many cases the test results showed little, if any, indication of deficit. In other patients the level was much below expectation, suggestive of considerable "impairment." This latter finding occurred most typically in patients with withdrawal types of reactions who failed to answer questions or to perform the required tasks so that their scores were necessarily low or zero. These patients might answer the first few items of a subtest, then fail to respond or just say "I don't know" to others. Thus one 11-year-old patient (Case 56) with an elementary school education defined a donkey as an "animal" and diamond as "jewelry," but then failed to respond when asked the definition of such words as apple, join, fur, nuisance and cushion. She nodded or smiled when urged to go on or asked if she knew the answer, but still failed to say anything. Her obtained IQ was only 67.

In most cases the patients did not show patterns of scatter on the subtests supposedly characteristic of "organic brain disease." Thus about half the patients did better on performance than on Verbal tests and many patients did relatively well on such tests as Block Design, Object Assembly and Digit Symbol which have been regarded as most sensitive to organic impairment.

There were certain patterns of qualitative behavior that occurred on the Wechsler-Bellevue similar to that noted clinically. On the Information test, for example, many patients showed behavior somewhat analogous to paraphasia in which the response, although incorrect, was related to the subject matter in a tangential fashion. Thus the capital of Italy was variously given as "Genoa," "Venice," "Sicily," "Milan," "Capri" and "Naples." In these cases the patients, when then asked to name the largest city in Italy, usually answered Rome, indicating that their misidentification of the capital was not merely a case of defective memory or unfamiliarity. Similarly, the capital of Denmark was given as "Hamlet" and that of Japan was given as "Hiroshima" or as "Shanghai" and "Nagasaki." This common substitutive naming of cities suggests that the patient is using the name in a personalized symbolic sense rather than simply exhibiting a defect in memory.

Other errors observed on this test include the naming of "Rickenbacker" and "Lindbergh" as inventors of the airplane, saying that Hamlet was written by "Julius Caesar" and "Huckleberry Finn" by "Tom Sawyer," locating Brazil in "Argentina" or "Mexico," attributing the discovery of the North Pole to "Marco Polo" or "Christopher Columbus," and stating that Washington's birthday was the "4th of July." On the question of the number of weeks in a year such responses were given as "48," "52 and sometimes 53," "56," and "52 weeks and 6 hours." We have been accustomed to referring to this pattern of response on the Information test as the "Genoa syndrome."

In many instances a patient received a lower score on the Wechsler-Bellevue because he used the question as a means of expressing some particular personal reference, usually connected with illness. Thus the explanation of why a marriage license was required was commonly given as "for health's sake" or "to prove you're in good health." One patient explained the similarity of the eye and the ear as "when you have a doctor—an eye, ear, nose and throat doctor—he looks through your ears and wants to know about your eyes." The function of the heart was explained as "when your heart isn't alright you're sick." One patient, asked what a thermometer was, said, "The greatest indignity in life is to have a rectal thermometer." Another, asked why laws are necessary, said, "To prevent doctors like you from asking so many questions." On the Picture Completion test, in which the patient is asked to tell what is missing, one woman remarked that a figure was "crippled" because he was walking with a cane. Sometimes the personal reference took a humorous form. A woman responded to a question about the population of the United States with "Male and Female?" Another when asked who discovered the North Pole, said, "It wasn't Mr. North." A depressed patient, without verbal denial, explained why we have taxes by "death and taxes, like it or not, we're going to have it."

Occasionally cryptic responses were used which likewise appeared to have a particular personalized meaning to the patient. These included defining the Vatican as a "religious present indication" and answering why shoes are made of leather with "as a rule when most people wear anything on their feet, they usually resort to leather."

Tests of memory were of particular interest in these patients because of the theories advanced by some writers of the role of loss of memory in the production of anosognosia, disorientation, and reduplication. On a formal test, such as the Wechsler Memory Scale, the scores obtained were at the same level as on the Wechsler-Bellevue Scale, indicating that memory was not better or worse than the general level of intellectual functioning. There was no difference between patients with verbal denial and those with implicit forms of denial.

A special study was made of patients who showed reduplication since Pick (1903) in calling it "reduplicative paramnesia" felt this phenomenon could be explained on the basis of a memory disturbance. For comparison, other patients with brain disease who showed some evidence of memory difficulty on routine clinical examinations were studied. No correlation was found between reduplication and scores on the Memory Scale. Actually, many of the patients with the lowest scores failed to show the phenomenon while some of the patients with reduplication had scores over 100.

The nature of the memory factors important in disorientation and denial was perhaps best brought out by a test involving recall of selected stories. Besides the two paragraphs on the Memory Scale, the patients were given two other brief stories to repeat. One had no reference to illness while the other was based on a fable and given to the patients as follows:

> There once was a king who was very sick and his doctors were unable to cure him. He sent for his wise men who told him he would get well if he wore the shirt of a truly happy man. He sent his messengers out all over the kingdom looking for a truly happy man and they finally found one, but he didn't have a shirt.

While the patients might have done well in their recall of other material, they did especially poorly on the "King story." This seemed to be mainly because of a selective factor as a result of which the king's illness was the particular aspect for which memory was poor. Examples of recall of the first part of the story are: "There was a happy man that had some sheep. They ran away from him and he couldn't find them." "Once upon a time there was a king. He was very, very well." "Once there was a kingdom that had a king who was very happy except that he didn't have a shirt." "It's about a man who wanted to live a very happy life."

From these observations it is apparent that the disturbance in memory found in patients with denial of illness is a selective, rather than a general impairment.

In the interpretation of proverbs there was also a great degree of selectivity. Patients were apt to interpret proverbs having to do with their personal problems in quite "concrete" fashion while others were translated into "abstract" terms quite satisfactorily. Thus when asked the meaning of "Empty barrels make the most noise" one man replied, "My head is an empty barrel," whereas he was able to make generalized applications of other proverbs.

Figure drawings were obtained in almost all cases. In the patients whose neurological disability was confined mainly to one side of the body, there was a pronounced

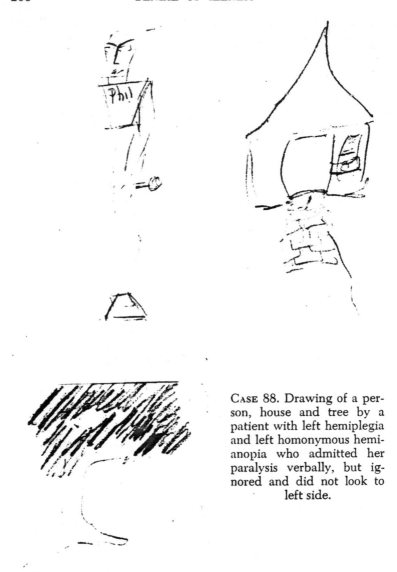

CASE 88. Drawing of a person, house and tree by a patient with left hemiplegia and left homonymous hemianopia who admitted her paralysis verbally, but ignored and did not look to left side.

tendency to asymmetry in their drawings. The omissions and distortions occurred on the side mirroring the patient's defect. Thus a patient with a left hemiplegia would draw a person with only one arm and one leg, with no extremities indicated on the left side of the page, although actually the right side of the person in the drawing. The asymmetry was likewise evident even in the drawings of a house or a tree in which windows might be left out on one side or the branches drawn only in one direction. The phenomenon of asymmetrical drawing occurred almost exclusively in patients who showed implicit forms of denial. Only two patients with explicit verbal denial omitted the limbs mirroring their hemiplegia. It thus appears that this behavior can be regarded primarily as another form of implicit denial. The patient who is able to deny his illness verbally draws a whole figure. In the other cases the omission of part

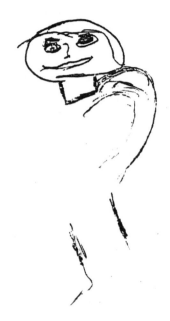

CASE 30. Drawing of a person by a patient with left hemiplegia and left homonymous hemianopia who explicitly denied paralysis and visual defect.

of a figure serves as another non-verbal device of avoiding or ignoring the reality of his illness. Some examples of this graphic form of implicit denial are shown in the figures.

On the Bender Visual Motor Gestalt test very few patients showed characteristics commonly regarded as occurring in brain disease such as rotation of the figure or alteration of the configuration. Mainly the behavior was within the limits to be found in a general hospital population. In some cases there was difficulty with one side of the figures comparable to that noted in the drawing test. This result is consistent with the tendency to do better on performance tests as shown on the Wechsler-Béllevue.

In their behavior on the Rorschach test there was also much variation in the type of records found. Some were of the order commonly described as occurring in brain disease, showing such features as few responses, perseveration and color naming. In other cases the results failed to show any evidence of "organic" impairment, according to the usual criteria. In most cases, however, there were aspects of behavior on the test comparable to that noted clinically. These included confabulation, condensation and inaccurate responses based on selective perception of only one aspect of the blot. There were also many responses symbolic of feelings of injury or damage to parts of the body.

The records obtained in patients with verbal denial of illness were compared with those in whom there were implicit forms of denial. From the anatomical and physiological point of view there should have been no differences between these groups since they had comparable pathology. But because of the importance of the pre-morbid personality certain significant differences would have been expected.

The results actually confirmed the latter hypothesis. The patients with explicit denial gave fewer responses, rejected more cards and showed a far greater poverty and stereotypy of content. They gave more whole and fewer small detail or space responses. Form was predominantly used as the sole determinant in this group, with little color, movement and shading. In the group with implicit denial, however, there were many movement, color and shading responses, and greater heterogeneity in the variety of responses. Sex, food and anal content were more frequent in these cases, as were responses with euphoric or paranoid implications.

Although in general the types of records found in the two groups were quite distinct, there was some overlapping in a few cases where the differentiation was not so clear. These were patients who likewise in their clinical behavior showed mixed forms of denial. The Rorschach results are considered, however, to support the importance of the pre-morbid personality as a factor in determining the pattern of denial shown.

Chapter X

EXPERIMENTAL PRODUCTION OF DENIAL

A NOSOGNOSIA in delusional form could be produced experimentally in certain patients with existing disabilities by altering the milieu of brain function. This was done pharmacologically with barbiturates and in more enduring fashion by means of a series of electrically induced convulsions.

EFFECTS OF BARBITURATES

It was noted that when apparently recovered patients who previously had shown denial of illness and disorientation were interviewed after an intravenous injection of amytal sodium, denial and disorientation were again expressed. Thus the patient (Case 3) whose disorientation and denial of operation and impotence was described in Chapter IV has been followed for several years. For a year after his discharge from the hospital he was completely oriented and admitted the fact of his operation, but when asked about his sexual impotence he would neither admit nor deny it saying often that he "hadn't tried to find out yet." He was given amytal sodium three weeks after disorientation had cleared and became disoriented for place stating that he was in a "hotel in Bad Nauheim, Germany, which is called Mount Sinai Hospital." He denied having had an operation. There was disorientation for time of day. On April 23 the procedure was repeated with 0.5 gms. of amytal. He named the

110

hospital correctly but placed it in Mainz, Germany, later in Portugal, and also made references to being in "San Diego Hospital" and a restaurant. He admitted having an operation but said it had been on his back. There was only slight disorientation for time of day.

After discharge from the hospital, the patient returned in June of 1949 for a revision of the bone flap. On June 22 0.45 gms. of amytal sodium were given intravenously. The patient confabulated that he had just taken a trip to see a friend who lived in another part of the city but there were no other manifestations of disorientation. In May, 1950 the patient was readmitted for the insertion of a tantalum plate as he had complained of headaches. The patient still had a visual field defect of which he did not complain but he was depressed, and for the first time expressed great anxiety over his continued impotence. The administration of 0.5 gms. of intravenous amytal on this occasion yielded no evidence at all of disorientation or denial of any of his difficulties.

Similarly, in patients with brain disease who on clinical examination show no evidence of altered behavior, an interview with amytal sodium may produce verbal denial and disorientation. An example of this and the technic of administration is provided by the patient whose behavior was described in Chapter III (Case 54). The patient not only became disoriented and denied illness under the influence of the drug, but showed much of the ludic behavior that he was to display later in his illness. Prior to receiving the drug he was completely oriented and admitted headache, poor vision and loss of libido and sexual potency. The following protocol was recorded shortly after his admission to the hospital. A solution of 0.5 gms. in 10 cc. of water was used.

Time elapsed from start of injection		*Amount*
1'00"	.... (Patient counting backward)	0.05 gm.
2'50"	.... (Errors in counting backward)	0.15 gm.
4'10"	.... (Nystagmus appeared)	0.2 gm.

EXAMINER	PATIENT
What do you call this place?	I have no idea.
How long have you been here?	Two or three days.
What sort of a place is it?	No.
Does it have a name?	(No answer.)
Why are you here?	To sell furniture.
Any other reason?	No.
Name of this place?	No idea.
Anything the matter with you?	No.
Sick?	No.
Perfectly well?	Yes, sir.
Been in a hospital recently?	(No answer.)
Time now?	7:20 (actually 4:00 p.m.).
Morning or evening?	Evening.
Had Supper?	No.
Today's date?	Thursday, September 20, 1920.
How old are you?	Twenty-one.
When were you born?	Jan. 16, 1901 (correct).
Anything the matter with your eyes?	Definitely.
What?	Poor sight.
What is it due to?	Drinking.
Any headaches?	No.
Any sexual difficulty?	No.
When did you have intercourse last?	Two to three months ago (probably a confabulation).
Where?	Chicago.
Where is this place?	Have no idea—all the way up in the heart of the district.

EXAMINER	PATIENT
How far from your home is this place?	Three miles (distance of patient's business address from his home).
12'15" (needle removed)	
What do I do here?	You're a doctor.
What do you call this place?	An average lay-in hospital
What's it for?	For people who have things done for them and so on and so forth.
Why are you here?	I'm going to have a baby.
How can you have a baby?	Doing the reverse English.
Where does the baby come from?	Right here (indicates abdomen).
I think you are kidding	Well, I can't help that—do you really?
Where is this place?	Just below where I live—in the William Penn Hotel.
What street?	I don't know—give me a cigarette.
What time is it now?	7:00 (actually 4:10).
Have you had headaches?	No.
What is the name of this hospital?	Pittsburgh General.
What city?	Pittsburgh.
Pittsburgh?	I hope so.
Why are you in the hospital?	To give birth.
Isn't that unusual?	Not my way (patient is restless).
What time is it now?	8:00.
Isn't it light for 8:00?	Well, we are west of the Alleghonies. I've seen you before.
Where?	On the furniture market.
But I'm a doctor.	There are lots of doctors on the furniture market.
Why did you come to the hospital?	To prove I'm innocent.
Of what?	Of attacking a girl.
Do you know where you are now?	Pittsburgh.
Time now?	7:30.

At 5:00 p.m. nystagmus was no longer present. The patient named the hospital correctly, located it within

10 blocks of its actual site, gave the correct date and time and admitted all aspects of his illness without confabulation.

One week later the patient received 9.0 cc. of normal saline intravenously and the routine "amytal" prooeduro was carried out. There was no change in orientation, no denial of illness, no misidentification or confabulation.

After the patient's discharge from the hospital, he showed no overt behavior disturbances although his EEG record remained abnormal. One year later the "amytal test" was repeated using 0.45 gms. of the drug. He became markedly disoriented for place (Carleton Terrace) and denied ever having had headaches or sexual difficulty.

USE OF THE AMYTAL TEST IN THE DIAGNOSIS OF BRAIN DISEASE

Inasmuch as such patterns of denial and disorientation were shown only in patients with existing brain damage, this procedure has been useful in establishing the presence of brain disease. The elicitation on repeated questioning of verbal denial of illness or disorientation for place expressed as verbal identification, condensation, displacement, misnaming and the confabulated journey occurred only in patients with demonstrable brain damage. Similarly normal persons did not persistently confuse day and night or become disoriented for year. The procedure given at successive stages of the illness has also been helpful in evaluating the course and prognosis.

Normal persons while not directly denying illness or becoming disoriented showed many of the other alterations in language described in Chapter VI. They frequently talked about their illness in the *third person* whereas prior to receiving the drug they had described their symptoms in the first person. Thus a patient in the preliminary interview answered the question "Are you worried" with

"No, I ain't, it's no use, I try to keep it off my mind." After receiving the drug, his reply to the same question was "Yes about my mother, she's been pretty sick, and my father hasn't been feeling well. Brother has stomach trouble and sister had scarlatina." A patient with a problem of alcoholism told during the drug injection how worried his mother was because his brother drank. Frequently a third person became the subject of the sentence where previously the patient had recounted the circumstances of his illness in the first person. Thus, "I want to go home" was changed to "My family wants me to go home." Or a patient who, prior to getting the drug, said "I have diabetes" substituted *"They* told me I have diabetes." Other changes found in normals were paraphasic misnaming, misinterpretation of questions having to do with illness and hospitalization, and the use of slang, humor and metaphor.

EFFECTS OF ELECTRIC SHOCK

Another means of creating a change in the state of brain function was by the administration of electric shock convulsions. Opportunities to observe its effects came when twelve patients with intractable pain were treated in an attempt to obtain relief. The repeated production of typical patterns of verbal denial and displacement, disorientation, various forms of reduplication and paraphasia and the occurrence of a marked *"abstinence syndrome"* makes a detailed account of the following case significant:

A 48-year-old housewife, was admitted to the neurological service in The Mount Sinai Hospital on April 28, 1950 because of pain and progressive weakness in her legs. On May 5 a hemangioma was removed from the spinal cord at the T8 level. As she did not improve following this procedure, a second laminectomy was performed on June 27 and an extensive arachnoiditis reported. After this

operation the patient developed a complete paraplegia in
flexion with severe deformity, and a bed sore. There was
marked diminution of all sensory modalities below the T8
dermatome and she had urinary and fecal retention. She
complained of increasingly severe pain in her legs un-
relieved by codeine, demerol, and methadone. The patient
was depressed, bitter, and irritable, would scream in
agonized fashion, and would reproach the staff for not
responding more sympathetically to her.

On October 1, 1950 a course of ECT using the Reiter
apparatus was begun in an effort to control her pain. She
was given three treatments on consecutive days. Several
hours after the second treatment she seemed more hostile
and suspicious toward the nurses than heretofore and
refused to let them touch her legs. She asked, "What happened to my legs; they are bent . . . they were never that
way before." She repeatedly asked if she had just awakened from a dream. The expressed feeling of unfamiliarity with her surroundings was striking. Following the third
treatment the patient became affable, no longer complained of pain, and in an interview on October 4 denied
having any pain even on direct questioning. When she
was asked why she was in the hospital she replied, "My
feet won't walk." She remarked on "how nice everyone is
to me" and joked with the staff. She was disoriented for
place, naming the hospital correctly but placing it in another part of the city. She was also disoriented for date
naming the month as September or April. She believed
that she had been in the hospital only two months. On
several occasions she was disoriented for the time of day.
In naming objects she made paraphasic errors, such as
calling a tongue blade a "ruler." An EEG performed on
October 6 showed diffuse delta activity at a frequency
of 3 to 6 per second.

The state of affability lasted for three days during
which no further shocks were given. She then began to
complain of pain again, reproaching the nurses in a queru-
lous fashion. She was only slightly disoriented for time

and place and showed no paraphasia. She was given an injection of 0.2 gms. of amytal sodium and while under the influence of the drug she denied pain in her legs and complained of pain only in her arm, at the site of the injection. She also became more markedly disoriented for time and place.

On October 9 shock treatments were resumed and she was given nine convulsions on consecutive days. At the end of the series she was again euphoric and did not complain of pain even though she was observed to wince when turning in bed. When catheterized she moaned as if in pain but joked with the doctors. She showed a reduplicative disorientation for place, claiming that she had come from "another Mount Sinai Hospital" situated nearby. She stated that each hospital had the same doctors and nurses but that in the "other Mount Sinai Hospital" the nurses had been very inconsiderate. "You could yell your guts out and get nowhere." In the present hospital, however, the nurses were described as "kind and wonderful."

The state of elation lasted for two days and she then became disturbed, hyperactive and paranoid. She refused medication for fear she would be poisoned. When an examiner moved her leg she asked, "What are you trying to do, place it back on me?" While her catheter was being changed she asked if she were having a miscarriage. This behavior lasted for one week and on October 23 the patient appeared rational and again complained of pain. She was well oriented and named objects correctly and interpreted her experience as a bad dream. She explained that she had thought that the room opposite her (patients' sitting room) was a whorehouse and that the nurses were trying to kill her. She thought that the side rails on her bed had grown thinner and this was a sign that she was going to die. She also said that she believed that the trouble with her legs had occurred because she had allowed a friend to perform cunnilingus on her.

During the next three weeks she became increasingly anxious and complained of a great deal of pain. She remained completely oriented and the EEG showed only a small degree of abnormality. Amytal sodium given intravenously produced only a slight transient disorientation with no denial of pain. She was depressed, cried and pleaded for injections to make her sleep. On November 15 a third course of ECT was begun with the development of much the same course of events shown previously. After the 11th treatment, she became euphoric, showed a reduplicative disorientation for place, stating that she was in a hospital near her home, to which she referred as the "younger Mount Sinai." She was also disoriented for time of day and gave paraphasic naming responses as calling a hypodermic needle a "tiepin." She claimed that her foot, which in its flexion deformity rested on her thigh, was the examiner's hand. She demanded that it be taken away but, although she kept complaining, began to joke about it and remarked that if the hand were not removed she would lose her virginity and would have to redivorce her husband.

The euphoric period was a brief one, lasting only a few hours, and the patient again became agitated and paranoid. She said that her legs had been pasted together by the examiner's brother. Another shock treatment was given and the next day she was again affable. However, on the same day she became agitated, complained of pain, and expressed a fear of dying. She thought the nurses were trying to poison her and telephoned the police to save her. She begged repeatedly to be put to sleep. She expressed the idea that her deformed legs were a kind of animal in her bed with her and asked, "Why do I have two assholes?" referring to a bedsore that had developed. She broke a candy jar and after threatening to slash a nurse, tried to cut her own wrist with a fragment.

One week later she was rational, clearly oriented and complained of severe pain. She explained that she had gotten the idea that, while smoking in bed, she had burned down the "old Mount Sinai Hospital" with the patients and that she was being killed for this in the "New Mount Sinai." Although she now knew that this was not true she asked to be reassured that she hadn't burned down the hospital. When asked why she had tried to kill herself she answered, "I didn't want to kill myself. All I wanted to do was to go to sleep. I thought I could do this by pulling blood out of a vein and counting, just like when the doctors did it to me." The patient apparently was referring to the injections of pentothal sodium that were given prior to each treatment.

The premorbid personality suggested that a paranoid form of denial would develop. She was described by her relatives as an impulsive and excitable person who usually was good natured but who had a quick temper. She was energetic in a restless way and kept house in a slipshod manner. She had always been frightened of illness, pain, and hospitals, but was not a complainer. In the present illness she seemed to get temporary relief from pain by screaming and yelling. She was extremely sympathetic and generous to people who were ill or in trouble and would be hurt if others did not respond similarly to her. She would try to cover up this sensitivity, however, by appearing "hard" and flippant. She had been bitter that friends had not visited her in the hospital and when they did come, she berated them severely, then carried on with the visit in a friendly fashion. She was stubborn and headstrong and, if she did not get her own way, was likely to have a tantrum. She was not an openly warm and affectionate person but made friends and liked company. She had married at 19, had four children, and was divorced at 33 after she had become involved with "fast company." Following the divorce she drank heavily for a while "to forget her troubles" but liquor generally made her "feel sorry for herself."

A patient with dystonia musculorum deformans who complained of pain in her neck was also treated with electric shock. After the seventh convulsion she no longer complained of pain and appeared untroubled by her deformity and bizarre gait. Formerly she had been self-conscious and refused to leave her room but now she walked about openly. She attributed others looking at her to a sexual interest. During this period the patient expressed reduplication for place, person and time. Another patient with dystonia and pain received the same number of electrically induced convulsions but did not develop disorientation nor did she deny her deformity or pain. Others received as high as 18 convulsions without developing disorientation, paraphasia or reduplication, even with the use of amytal sodium. It was only in patients who showed such alterations in symbolic expression that apparent relief from pain was accomplished.

Case 38 was that of a man with a sub-frontal meningioma who denied blindness and operation in a euphoric, paranoid manner. From the history, it was learned that four years prior to hospitalization, he had been depressed, had become sexually impotent and had expressed paranoid feelings about members of his family. At that time he was institutionalized and received a course of ECT and insulin treatment. Following these he was said to have recovered completely. His family described him as cheerful, unworried and unconcerned with any problems. This euphoric state lasted for one year. It is likely that the patient's symptoms were related to his brain tumor and that altering the conditions of brain function iatrogenically, permitted the development of a syndrome of denial, comparable to that shown subsequently after the tumor had progressed.

These findings suggest that the therapeutic effect of ECT may be related to the production of a state of brain function in which patterns of denial may operate. The type of denial that is expressed is in large part determined

by the character of the premorbid personality. At present
we are investigating the relationship among clinical
changes in behavior following ECT, personality factors
and the symbolic patterns elicited under amytal sodium,
at various stages during the treatment.

It is likely that the changes in brain function sufficient
for the existence of anosognosia may be produced by
many other physiological, pharmacological and mechanical agents. The denial of failing capacities and the exaggerated opinion of one's ability that may occur in states
of anoxemia is an example. Alcohol and cortisone as well
as barbiturates may also act in this fashion. We have observed several patients with neurological deficit who during the period of treatment with cortisone became euphoric and insisted that they were better, although there was
no objective change in the extent of disability. Inasmuch
as cortisone is produced as part of a normally occurring
physiological process, the study of alterations in the language of patients receiving it is of particular importance.

Chapter XI

SUMMARY AND THEORETICAL
CONSIDERATIONS

THE review of the more than 50 years of study of the problem of denial of illness indicates that the observer's concept of anosognosia, his interpretation of the anatomical and physiological data, his ideas of what constitute adequate methods of study, and his acceptance of the proof of a particular theory were determined in large part by certain a priori concepts. Thus, if anosognosia is regarded as a unitary defect of "body scheme" one is concerned mainly with demonstrating a loss of perception or recognition of the affected part of the body. If one "knows" that a particular form of anosognosia is "caused" by a lesion in the parietal lobe or the thalamus then the finding of a lesion involving either structure constitutes "proof" of the validity of the idea. The observer is then apt to disregard not only other manifestations of altered behavior but to dismiss the importance of lesions in other areas actually found at autopsy.

Historically, the tendency has been to divide forms of denial of illness into artificial units of behavior. This has been manifested, for example, by a classification in terms of the particular symptom or defect that is denied. Denial of hemiplegia, denial of blindness and lack of concern over illness have been treated as separate entities involving dysfunction of different areas of the brain. While one observer may approach a patient with anosognosia for hemiplegia from the standpoint of a defect in "body scheme" and a parietal lobe lesion, another may consider a patient who expresses denial by joking unconcern about illness from the view of "loss of insight" or impairment of "abstract attitude" relating to frontal lobe pathology.

Our findings indicate that the various forms of anosognosia are not discrete entities that can be localized in different areas of the brain. Whether a lesion involves the frontal or parietal lobe determines the disability that may be denied, not the mechanism of denial. Thus the patterns of anosognosia for hemiplegia and blindness do not differ from those in which the fact of an operation or the state of being ill is denied. Under the requisite conditions of brain function the patient may deny the paralysis of an arm whether it results from a fracture, an injury to the brachial plexus, a brain stem or a cortical lesion. The effect of the brain damage is to provide the milieu of altered function in which the patient may deny *anything* that he feels is wrong with him. Some motivation to deny illness and incapacity exists in everyone and the level of brain function determines the particular perceptual-symbolic organization, or language, in which it is expressed. The phenomena of verbal denial, disorientation, reduplication and "paraphasia" are not individual defects that can be directly represented in anatomical or physiological terms. They are rather examples of such integrations of language. The same anatomical and physiological conditions subserve not only the verbal forms of denial but many other forms of symbolic adaptation. The fact that one patient may express an explicit denial and another show a withdrawn akinetic state or altered sexual behavior is related not to differently located lesions but to features in the premorbid personality.

In regarding these phenomena as modes of adaptation to stress rather than as individual defects it should be pointed out that they were in large measure products of a particular environmental situation. The group of environmental factors included not only the level of brain function, but the patient's disability, the hospital milieu and his past experience. Thus the various patterns of denial were elicited usually by specific questions and conditions in a particular interpersonal situation. Thus disorientation for place generally cleared when the patient went home. Paraphasia was commonly manifested only when the patient named objects connected with his illness or some personal problem. While a patient might show "loss of insight" in relation to his illness, his judgment in other areas might be excellent. Alterations of sexual behavior usually appeared in the patients' relationship to a doctor or nurse rather than to another patient or a visitor. One of us (Kahn and Schlesinger, 1951) has reported the case of a patient whose disorientation and fecal and urinary incontinence cleared promptly when he went home. While such a dramatic change is uncommon it illustrates the importance of environmental factors. In evaluating the effect of brain damage on behavior it is important that it not be done on the basis of an examination at a single time or in a single situation. The patient should serve as his own control and his behavior should be observed in comparable interpersonal situations at different times and places and if possible under varying conditions of brain function.

The problem of how these multiple environmental factors are integrated remains to be solved. The changes in brain function appeared to affect the *pattern* rather than the *elements* of the symbolic expression of denial. Thus patients who had hitherto tended to use verbal forms of denial tended to develop a verbal anosognosia while those who had previously relied on other modes of adaptation persisted in them. Pattern refers here to the spatial and temporal organization of the language of denial. The pat-

terns of disorientation and reduplication occurred repeatedly and uniformly in patient after patient. The particular name or person that was used was determined by the
patient's own experience, while its mode of integration
depended on the level of brain function. Prior to becoming disoriented, the patient spoke of his wish to go home
and be well. In the phase of disorientation, he expressed
the same motivation by misnaming the hospital, "moving" it closer to his home or confabulating that he had left
the hospital. The integration of the same symbolic element into various patterns at changing levels of brain
function was well seen in the case of the patient who
talked about the fictitious "Coolidge Memorial Hospital."
During the period of greatest alteration of brain function
he said that he "was" in "Coolidge Memorial." He then
confabulated that his friend had been there. When brain
function had further improved he was completely oriented
in a clinical sense but said he had the feeling that there
"must" be a Coolidge Memorial somewhere.

When the patient denies the paralysis of an arm, there
appears to be not simply an "imperception" of the limb
but a re-organization of perception in which the usual
temporal and spatial unities are superseded. When he
says that the arm belongs to the doctor or nurse or calls
the arm "he," "she" or "it," the patient seems to regard
himself and his arm as separate entities. Similarly, he does
not differentiate his having moved the arm in the past and
the hope of moving it in the future from movement in
the present. The ill person may say to the doctor "you
look sick, why don't you lie down." In reduplication, single entities are split into multiple parts while in condensation the patient "combines" two places into one. The
place or object that is misnamed no longer seems to have
a discrete existence of its own but is merged into the patient's feeling about himself. Thus the patient with a

tracheotomy and a paraparesis referred to the hospital as
"Fresh Air Roller Skating Academy," while a severely incapacitated man called a syringe "an old used radio
tube." There is thus a multifactorial system that includes
the patient's motivation, his particular symbolic values
and an organization of perception which enables the patient to express his motivation in terms of selected aspects
of the environment.

Our findings are related to some of the problems of
prefrontal lobotomy. This procedure when performed bilaterally evidently creates a milieu of brain function sufficient for the existence of anosognosia. After the operation patients may show all aspects of the syndrome of
denial: denial of the operation, disorientation, reduplication, confabulation, paraphasic language, mood changes
and urinary incontinence. The success or failure of the procedure seems to be a matter of what type of denial is expressed by the patient, and to some degree, by his doctor.
Thus, when explicit verbal denial of all problems is used
or when the patient is smilingly indifferent and says he is
getting along perfectly, then the result is regarded as
"successful." When the adaptation is one of apathy, rest-
lessness, extreme neglect of his person or alteration in
sexual behavior, then the outcome is considered as "unsuccessful." Usually the postoperative changes in behavior have been disregarded either as manifestations of
"confusion" or as complications of the operation. Relevant
observations are regarded as beginning only when the
patient is able to cooperate in formal testing. The generally negative findings on psychological tests after lobotomy
should make it clear that the behavior cannot be understood in terms of "defects." It may be precisely the "complications" which furnish the clue to the understanding
of the altered behavior.

The behavior seen in anosognosia is not peculiar to patients with brain disease but has much in common with symbolic modes of expression used under normal conditions of brain function. For example in dreaming, there is an interrelationship among an altered level of brain function, symbolic patterns and elements and motivations comparable to those of the ill person. In both sleep and the brain damaged patient there is a state of function characterized by a slowing of the EEG rhythm which under certain conditions may serve as the milieu for the expression of certain motivations in a particular mode of thought or action. In each state spatial and temporal modalities, persons, places, objects and even parts of the body may serve as symbols of some wish or need or feeling.

The observations of patients with denial is also helpful in appreciating the significance of certain types of behavior in young children. Thus confabulations about the "good mother" and the "bad mother" and the imaginary companion are reduplications in which the fictitious person is the symbolic representation of some need or feeling of the child. Children often talk of themselves in the third or second person and confabulate reports of the acts of others which are actually their own experience. An interesting instance of denial is cited by Sullivan in the probably apocryphal story of the boy who was caught getting into the jam. When faced with the crime, the child said, "I didn't touch the jam, my hand did." Paraphasic naming is frequent as in a child calling a dachshund a "bureau dog" or himself a "cowboy" because he is wearing a cowboy hat. It is of interest that recent studies in young children by Bender, Fink and Green (1953) have shown a type of perceptual organization in response to multiple stimuli similar to that commonly found in adults with brain disease.

Piaget (1951) has pointed out the significance of these

forms of language and play in young children as a symbolic system whereby the threatening aspects of reality
may be resolved. He cites the symbolic play relating to the
excretory functions of the body. At one year and nine
months, the child put one open box on another, sat on it
and said, "sitting on pot." Later her dolls dirtied themselves and at three and a half the feces were compared
paraphasically to a finger, a mouse, and a rabbit and given
ladies' names. A study of these symbolic patterns in relation to the development of perceptual organization in
children should be of value.

Piaget also raises the question as to whether the child
really believes his play is real. He feels that the two to
four-year-old does not stop to consider whether his ludic
representations are real or not. Similarly, in the patient
with anosognosia the need to avoid catastrophe is so over-
whelming that he seems not to think in terms of truth or
falsehood or logic or illogic but only in terms of survival
or destruction. If a discrepancy is noted it is probably disregarded as trivial or inconsequential. He operates in an
hedonic system of belief where what gives relief or satisfaction is "true" and what causes unhappiness is "false."

These considerations are of heuristic value because they
determine to what degree the observations concern the
interrelationship of motivation and neural organization in
all symbolic functions. If anosognosia is regarded as a
fixed defect caused by a focal brain lesion, then it can
have only a limited application to the behavior and language of normal persons. Edward Sapir (1934) has shown
that all language is patterned, involving a process of selective perception and generalization. The same articula-
tory and phonetic elements are used in one pattern for
referential communication and in another for the expression of other motivations. In poetry, prayer, drama, myth,
humor and slang, the mechanisms of reduplication, para-

phasia and disorientation appear. In brain disease the symbolic level tends to become rigid, fixed and enduring. Under normal conditions there is a constant interplay among various symbolic systems. All of these forms of language, whether occurring in people with brain disease or in the normal provide important forms of adaptation to the stresses of human existence.

TABLE 1
CLINICAL, NEUROLOGICAL, PATHOLOGICAL AND BEHAVIORAL DATA IN CASES WITH EXPLICIT DENIAL OF ILLNESS

Case No., Sex, Age	Lesion	Neurological Findings	Spinal Fluid	Electroencephalogram	Behavior
1 F 47	Spongioblastoma in right frontal lobe, extending deep to third ventricle; operation	Papilledema; staggering gait; urinary and fecal incontinence	Xanthochromic; pressure 280 mm. of water; total protein 100 mg./100 cc.	Diffuse delta activity; frequency 1-6 per sec., mainly in left frontal region	Denial of operation, urinary and fecal incontinence and illness; disorientation for place and time; euphoric, facetious and drowsy; displacement to third person; neologisms
2 M 47	Metastatic adenocarcinoma in right fronto-parietal region; operation	Papilledema; left hyper-reflexia and Babinski sign; urinary incontinence	Clear; pressure 180 mm. of water; total protein 49 mg./100 cc.	Diffuse delta activity; frequency 1-4 per sec., mainly from right inferior frontal electrode	Denial of operation and urinary incontinence; disorientation for date and place; affable, facetious; hallucinations
3 M 33	Chromophobe adenoma of pituitary; operation	Homonymous defect in lower right quadrant of visual fields; history of sexual impotence	Bloody after operation; pressure 260 mm. of water	Diffuse delta activity; 6 per sec.	Denial of operation, impotence; affable; disoriented for place and time
4 M 22	Chorioepithelioma of third ventricle invading right thalamus	Polyuria; polydipsia; bitemporal hemianopia; blindness fol-	Xanthochromic; pressure 105 mm. of water; total	Diffuse 3-6 per sec. activity	Denial of blindness and operation; hallucinations; disorientation for time and

130

	Pathology / Operation	Neurological findings	Cerebrospinal fluid	Electroencephalogram	Mental findings
	and internal capsule; operation; autopsy	lowing craniotomy	protein 180 mg./100 cc.		place; restless, drowsy, stereotyped movements
5 F 42	Piloid astrocytoma involving thalami, basal ganglia and corpus callosum; autopsy	Paralysis right leg; paresis right arm; involuntary movements of right leg; dystaxia of right arm; urinary and fecal incontinence	Clear; pressure 140-180 mm. of water; up to 215 lymphocytes per cu. mm.	Diffuse 4-6 per sec. activity	Denial of right hemiparesis, involuntary movements of right leg and urinary incontinence; disorientation for time and place; euphoric, paranoid; hallucinations
6 F 28	Glioma obliterating third ventricle, extending from posterior commissure to optic chiasm into median nuclei of thalamus; lateral ventricles enlarged; aqueduct displaced; autopsy	Nystagmus; paralysis of right conjugate gaze; bilateral ataxia; urinary incontinence	Clear; pressure 185 mm. of water; total protein 100 mg./100 cc.	Not recorded	Denial of illness and urinary incontinence; euphoric and drowsy; disorientation for time and place; paraphasia
7 F 38	Spongioblastoma of right temporal lobe; operation	Papilledema; left hemiplegia; urinary incontinence	Clear; pressure 280 mm. of water; total protein 41 mg./100 cc.	Diffuse delta activity with slowest frequency at frontal electrodes particularly on right	Denial of left hemiplegia and operation; paranoid; disorientation for time and place; delusions about sex and food
8 M 51	Intracranial metastases; mass in chest shown roentgenographically; dilata-	Papilledema; ataxic gait; urinary incontinence	Clear; ventricular fluid under increased pressure	Symmetrical diffuse 2-6 per sec. activity	Denial of incontinence, memory loss, illness and headaches; disoriented for time and place; reduplication for

TABLE 1. (Continued)

Case No., Sex, Age	Lesion	Neurological Findings	Spinal Fluid	Electroencephalo-gram	Behavior
	tion of lateral and third ventricles in ventriculogram; no lesion apparent on exploration of posterior fossa				time; paraphasia; euphoric, lethargic, paranoid
9 F 61	Cholesteatoma of third ventricle extending to infiltrate right thalamus, basal ganglia and internal capsule; operation; autopsy	Bilateral optic atrophy; pupils sluggish to light; staggering gait; bilateral Babinski sign; urinary incontinence	Faintly xanthochromic; pressure 120 mm. of water	Diffuse symmetrical 3-6 per sec. activity	Denial of illness and urinary incontinence; euphoric, facetious; disorientation for place and time
10 M 44	Craniopharyngioma filling third ventricle; autopsy	History of impotence; urinary incontinence	Clear; pressure 130 mm. of water; total protein 53 mg./100 cc.	Diffuse symmetrical 3-6 per sec. activity	Denial of impotence, urinary incontinence and memory loss; paranoid; reduplication for place, person and time; delusions about sex, violence, food, money
11 M 24	Chromophobe adenoma (?) of pituitary; enlarged, eroded sella apparent in roentgenogram	Polyuria; polydipsia; history of impotence; optic atrophy; bitemporal hemianopia, followed by blind-	Clear; pressure 80 mm. of water; total protein 111 mg./100 cc.	Not recorded	Denial of blindness and impotence; paranoid; disorientation for place and time; hallucinations

Case	Pathology	Neurological symptoms	Cerebrospinal fluid	Electroencephalogram	Psychiatric findings
		ness; paralysis of upward gaze; loss of pupillary reaction to light; bilateral Babinski sign; urinary incontinence			
12 M 32	Tumor of third ventricle (?); mass intruding into mesial wall of left lateral ventricle shown in pneumoencephalogram; neoplasm not disclosed at craniotomy	Polyuria; polydipsia; bitemporal hemianopia, followed by blindness; pupils fixed to light	Clear; pressure 110 mm. of water; total protein 200 mg./100 cc.	Diffuse 6-7 per sec. activity	Denial of blindness and operation; disorientation for time and place; euphoric, paranoid, lethargic
13 M 52	Acoustic neurinoma; cyst adherent to cerebellum; operation	Ataxic gait; nystagmus; deafness in right ear; anesthesia of right cornea	Clear; ventricular fluid under increased pressure	Not recorded	Denial of operation, memory loss; euphoric, paranoid; disorientation for time and place
14 M 48	Cholesteatoma of lateral ventricles; operation	Left hemiparesis; urinary incontinence	Xanthochromic; pressure 110 mm. of water	Diffuse 4-6 per sec. activity	Denial of left hemiparesis, operation; disorientation for time and place; euphoric, depressed
15 F 42	Neoplasm of midbrain (?); dilatation and asymmetry of lateral and third ventricles and displacement to left of caudal part of third ventricle shown	Papilledema; paresis of upward gaze; rigidity of all extremities; urinary incontinence	Xanthochromic; pressure 380 mm. of water	Diffuse symmetrical 3-6 per sec. activity	Denial of operation, illness and death of parents; disorientation for time and place; reduplication for time, person and place; euphoric, paranoid; hallucinations

TABLE 1. (Continued)

Case No., Sex, Age	Lesion	Neurological Findings	Spinal Fluid	Electroencephalogram	Behavior
	in ventriculogram; no tumor revealed on exploration of posterior fossa				
16 M 58	Chromophobe adenoma of pituitary; operation	Optic atrophy; bitemporal hemianopia; blindness; urinary and fecal incontinence	Clear; pressure 110 mm. of water; total protein 95 mg./100 cc.	Not recorded	Denial of operation, illness, blindness; disorientation for time and place; hallucinations; lethargic
17 F 47	Sarcoma of left orbit invading anterior fossa; operation	No preoperative symptoms; incontinence of urine after operation	Bloody after operation	1-2 per sec. delta activity over both frontal areas	Denial of operation, urinary incontinence and illness; euphoric, facetious; disorientation for time and place; reduplication for person and place; paraphasia
18 M 59	Transitional glioma of left frontal lobe; operation	Ataxic gait; papilledema; bilateral Babinski sign; urinary incontinence	Xanthochromic; pressure 230 mm. of water; total protein 280 mg./100 cc.	Normal record	Denial of operation and illness; jovial, facetious; disorientation for time and place; hallucinations
19 F 41	Intracranial (?) metastasis from adenocarcinoma of sig-	Grand mal convulsion; slight left hemiparesis	Clear; pressure 170 mm. of water; total protein 78	Diffuse 6-7 per sec. delta activity	Denial of operation, illness and fecal incontinence; euphoric; paraphasia; redup-

134

moid (laparotomy)		mg./100 cc.	Not recorded	lication for place; disorientation for time and place
20 M 56	Acoustic neurinoma; operation	Ataxic gait; nystagmus; deafness in right ear; absence of right corneal reflex; urinary incontinence	Clear; pressure 180 mm. of water; total protein 240 mg./100 cc.	Not recorded	Denial of operation and illness; bland, affable; disorientation for time and place; reduplication for time and place
21 M 53	Ependymoma of right lateral ventricle; operation	Papilledema; ataxic gait; urinary incontinence	Bloody after operation	Diffuse 4-6 per sec. delta activity	Denial of operation, incontinence of urine and sexual impotence; disorientation for time; misnaming of hospital; euphoric, paranoid; ludic behavior relating to work and money
22 F 40	Vascular anomaly of right temporo-parietal lobe; pineal shift down in angiogram	Left hemiparesis; left homonymous hemianopia; papilledema; retinal hemorrhage	Xanthochromic; pressure 120 mm. of water	Diffuse 6 per sec. delta activity	Denial of illness and memory loss; euphoric, facetious, apathetic; disorientation for time and place; pain asymbolia
23 F 35	(?) Left hemiplegia during pelvic infection following abortion in sixth month of pregnancy	Left hemiplegia and left sided sensory loss	Clear; pressure 120 mm. of water; total protein 35 mg./100 cc.	Diffuse 2-6 per sec. activity bilaterally; slower on right side	Denial of hemiplegia with displacement of arm into space, pelvic infection and death of baby; disorientation for time and place; reduplication for place, time and person; hallucinations; euphoric, depressed; paraphasia
24	Subfrontal meningto-	History of convulsion;	Clear; normal pres-	Diffuse 3-6 per sec.	Denial of operation, convul-

TABLE 1. (Continued)

Case No., Sex, Age	Lesion	Neurological Findings	Spinal Fluid	Electroencephalogram	Behavior
F 52	ma compressing optic chiasm; craniotomy	bilateral anosmia; marked impairment of vision postoperatively; incontinence of urine	sure; protein 192 mg./100 cc.	activity, particularly in frontal regions	sions and visual loss; disorientation for place, time of day; paraphasia; euphoric, paranoid; hallucinations
25 F 34	Metastases to brain of carcinoma of breast; previous mastectomy	Dysphasia; finger dysgnosia; dyscalculia; left right disorientation; weakness of left upper extremity; left Horner's syndrome	Not done	Diffuse delta activity, slowest frequencies at left inferior frontal, inferior parietal and ear lobe electrodes and right parieto-occipital leads	Denial of aphasia, operation and death of husband and son; paranoid; disorientation for time and place; paraphasia (?)
26 M 21	Brain injury; subarachnoid bleeding; traumatic amputation of left arm and fracture of jaw	No focal signs	Bloody, then clear	Diffuse slowing, chiefly in right occipital region (⅜ to 3 per sec.)	Denial of amputation; head and eyes averted to right; lethargic, restless; disorientation for place, time; paraphasia
27 F 47	Aneurysm of circle of Willis; subarachnoid hemorrhage; angiogram; craniotomy	Neck rigidity; incontinence of urine	Xanthochromic; pressure 110 mm. of water; protein 85 mg./100 cc.	Diffuse bilateral 4-6 per sec. activity with superimposed high voltage bursts	Denial of operations and illness; reduplication for place and time; disorientation for place and time; euphoric, depressed; paraphasia; hallucinations

136

	Diagnosis	Clinical findings	Spinal fluid	EEG	Psychiatric findings
28 F 57	Glioblastoma of frontal lobes; craniotomy; pneumoencephalogram showed displacement of left lateral and third ventricles	History of memory loss and headache; slight weakness in right upper extremity	Clear fluid; pressure 280 mm. of water; total protein 143 mg./100 cc.	Diffuse delta activity with frequencies as low as 0.8 per sec. at left frontal, temporal and right frontal, temporal, central and ear lobe electrodes	Denial of operation and death of mother; reduplication for person; disorientation for time and place; bland, cheerful mood; paraphasia
29 M 23	Bullet wound through right frontal region; craniotomy; cranioplasty	Skull defect and history of prolonged period of coma following injury	Normal	Minimal slowing in right anterior temporal region	Denial of having been wounded or of having had craniotomy; bland, affable
30 M 46	Cerebral hemorrhage with subarachnoid bleeding	Left hemiplegia and sensory loss; left homonymous hemianopia; incontinence of urine	Bloody	Diffuse slow wave activity as low as 1.8 per sec.; focal accentuation in right frontal region	Denial of hemiplegia and visual field defect; denial of being older than wife and that parents were dead; paranoid; disorientation for place and time; reduplication for time; altered sexual behavior
31 M 52	Metastatic carcinoma; marked swelling of right hemisphere; tumor masses in right frontal, right parieto-occipital and left frontal regions; craniotomy; autopsy	Left hemiparesis and sensory loss; bilateral papilledema with hemorrhage; incontinence of urine	Clear; pressure 260 mm. of water; total protein 112 mg./100 cc.	Diffuse slow activity at right frontal and parietal and left frontal electrodes	Denial of hemiplegia and illness; disorientation for place and time; reduplication for place; lethargic, restless, depressed; tragicludic; paraphasia

TABLE 1. (Continued)

Case No., Sex, Age	Lesion	Neurological Findings	Spinal Fluid	Electroencephalogram	Behavior
32 F 57	Softening of entire right cerebral hemisphere; herniation of right cingulate gyrus; carcinomatous metastases to liver and kidneys; autopsy	Left hemiplegia and sensory loss; right visual field defect; incontinence of urine	Clear; normal pressure; total protein 20 mg./100 cc.	Diffuse slow wave activity as low as 1.2 per sec. on all rightsided leads	Denial of hemiplegia; deviation of head and eyes to right; reduplication for place, time and parts of the body; disorientation for time; paraphasia
33 F 43	Subarachnoid hemorrhage; arteriography showed aneurysm of right internal carotid artery; ligation of common carotid artery	Stiff neck; ptosis of right upper eyelid; bilateral Babinskis; incontinence of urine and feces	Bloody then xanthochromic	Diffuse 1-3 per sec. activity	Denial of illness, death of sister and being unmarried; reduplication for place and person; disorientation for place and time; paraphasia
34 F 47	Probable aneurysm of circle of Willis	Weber's syndrome; right third nerve paralysis; left hemiplegia; incontinence of urine	Xanthochromic; normal pressure	Diffuse 2-3 per sec. activity	Denial of hemiplegia, ptosis, diplopia and being unmarried; reduplication for place and time; disorientation for place and time; affable; hallucinations; paraphasia
35 F 51	Subarachnoid hemorrhage; bilateral carotid angiography normal	Headache, stiff neck; history of hypertension; incontinence of urine and feces	Bloody then xanthochromic	Symmetrical bursts of 6 per sec. activity	Denial of illness and incontinence; disorientation for time and place; paraphasia; temporal reduplication; paranoid, depressed; hallucinations

138

	Diagnosis; operation	Clinical findings	CSF	EEG	Symptoms
36 F 53	Metastatic intracranial neoplasm of cerebellum; operation	Bilateral papilledema; dystaxia of right upper extremity; incontinence of urine	Not done	Symmetrical diffuse 4-6 per sec. activity with superimposed 2-3 per sec. bursts	Denial of operation and illness; reduplication for place, time and person; disorientation for time; euphoric, then depressed
37 F 46	Astrocytoma invading both frontal lobes; craniotomy; left frontal lobectomy	9 year history of convulsions	Not done	1.5 to 3 per sec. focus in left temporal lobe preoperatively; record not obtained postoperatively	Denial of illness, operation and convulsions; much displacement to third persons; disorientation for place and time; paraphasia; bland affect
38 M 32	Sub-frontal meningioma compressing optic chiasm; craniotomy	Bilateral papilledema; blindness complete in O.D., only light perception in O.S.; right pupil fixed to light; left pupil sluggish	Not done	Delta activity as low as 1 per sec. at all frontal electrodes	Denial of blindness and operation; disorientation for place; paraphasia; euphoric, paranoid
39 M 49	Occipital and basal skull fracture; laceration of brain	Right hemiparesis; right Babinski; previous enucleation of left eye	Bloody on admission, then clear	Diffuse not symmetrical 3-6 per sec. activity	Denial of hemiparesis, blindness and absence of left eye; reduplication for place, time and parts of the body; disorientation for time and place; paraphasia
40 M 59	Glioblastoma right hippocampal region; hemorrhagic encephalomalacia of thalami; autopsy	Left homonymous hemianopia; right Babinski; apraxia for dressing; weakness of left upper extremity	Clear; pressure 170 mm. of water; total protein 112 mg./100 cc.	Large amount of 2-6 per sec. activity at all right-sided electrodes	Denial of visual field defect and neglected left side; disorientation for time and place; vague, lethargic
41 F 46	Sphenoidal ridge meningioma compressing left tem-	Papilledema; mass over left temporal bone; right hemi-	Not done	Delta activity with frequencies as low as 1 per sec. at all	Denial of right hemiparesis; disorientation for place and time; lethargic, indifferent

TABLE 1. (Continued)

Case No., Sex, Age	Lesion	Neurological Findings	Spinal Fluid	Electroencephalo-gram	Behavior
	poral lobe	paresis; right hemi-sensory loss; dysphasia		electrodes, mostly in left ear lobe and inferior parie-tal leads	
42 M 47	Acoustic neurinoma; craniotomy followed by subarachnoid hemorrhage	Nystagmus; absent left corneal reflex; deaf-ness and dead laby-rinth on left; left peripheral facial paralysis	Preoperatively clear; postopera-tively bloody	Normal preopera-tively	Denial of operation and illness
43 F 38	Subarachnoid hemor-rhage; aneurysm of right and left internal carotid arteries on arteriography	Left hemiparesis and dysphasia following arteriogram; devel-oped flexion contrac-ture of legs; inconti-nence of urine and feces	Bloody then xanthochromic	Not done	Denial of hemiparesis, dys-phasia, incontinence and contractures; displacement to past and to third persons; reduplication for place and time; transient reduplica-tion of body parts; disorien-tation for place, time and person; paraphasia
44 M 59	Self-inflicted gunshot wound of frontal lobes; craniotomy	Skull defect; inconti-nence of urine and feces	Not done	4-6 per sec. activity over both frontal regions	Denial of injury, craniotomy and incontinence; disorien-tation for place and time; reduplication for place, time and person; affable, puerile, lethargic, apa-thetic; delusion that daugh-ter had a baby

140

Case	Diagnosis	Neurological signs	Spinal fluid	EEG	Psychiatric symptoms
45 F 22	Meningo-encephalitis	Retention and incontinence of urine; bilateral Babinski; myoclonic twitch of extremities; miotic sluggish pupils	Clear; 130 to 400 mm. of water pressure; 95 lymphocytes per cu. mm.; total protein 26 mg./100 cc.	Diffuse symmetrical activity from 1-6 per sec. with superimposed bursts	Denial of illness; reduplication for place and time; euphoric, hypomaniac, catatonic phases; altered sexual behavior; paraphasia, neologisms; disorientation for place and time; hallucinations
46 F 28	Glioblastoma right parieto-temporal region; herniation of right uncus and cingulate gyrus; craniotomy; autopsy	Slight left hemiparesis and left homonymous hemianopia; bilateral papilledema; incontinence of urine	Xanthochromic postoperatively	Diffuse 1-2 per sec. activity at all right-sided electrodes	Denial of illness, left hemiplegia and operation; displacement of illness and operation to minor area; disorientation for place and time; euphoric; paranoid, depressed; paraphasia
47 M 56	Glioblastoma of right frontal lobe extending into left frontal lobe and infiltrating basal ganglia and left lateral ventricl; autopsy	Bilateral papilledema; shuffling gait; ataxia of upper left extremity; incontinence of urine	Not done	Diffuse slow activity from 1.8 per sec. at both frontal and temporal electrodes	Denial of illness; disorientation for place; euphoric, depressed, lethargic
48 F 38	Brain stem neoplasm unverified; myelogram showed suggestive mass in foramen magnum; tracheotomy	Spastic paretic gait; nystagmus on lateral and upward gaze; fibrillation of tongue; dysphagia; old amputation of right arm; incontinence of urine	Clear; normal pressure; total protein 22 mg./100 cc.	Diffuse bisynchronous bursts of 5-6 per sec. activity prior to appearance of altered behavior	Denial of paraparesis, tracheotomy, illness and getting married; disorientation for place; euphoric, depressed; paraphasia
49 F 33	Occlusion of middle cerebral artery; rheumatic heart disease;	Left hemiplegia and left-sided sensory loss; left homony-	Not done	Diffuse slow wave activity from 1 per sec. over en-	Denial of hemiplegia and illness; disorientation for time of day; euphoric, jocu-

TABLE 1. (Continued)

Case No., Sex, Age	Lesion	Neurological Findings	Spinal Fluid	Electroencephalogram	Behavior
	auricular fibrillation	mous hemianopia		tire right hemisphere; small amount of slow activity on left	lar then depressed
50 F 58	Piloid astrocytoma of anterior portion of corpus callosum; craniotomy; autopsy	Incontinence of urine; bradykinesia	Not done	Delta activity as slow as 1 per sec. bilaterally at all frontal and left inferior parietal and ear lobe electrodes	Denial of operation, incontinence of urine and memory loss; disorientation for place and time; euphoric, depressed
51 F 58	Glioblastoma right temporal region; craniotomy	Left hemiparesis; left-sided sensory loss; left homonymous hemianopia; incontinence of urine	Clear fluid; pressure 160 mm. of water; total protein 60 mg./100 cc.	Diffuse delta activity as low as 0.7 per sec. over all right-sided electrodes and left frontal electrodes	Denial of operation and hemiparesis; reduplication for place and person; disorientation for time; euphoric; paraphasia
52 M 26	Bullet wound right fronto-parieto-occipital region; craniotomy	Skull defect; left hemiparesis; left dysstereognosis	Normal	Slow wave activity in right temporal, parietal, occipital leads	Denied having been wounded; reduplication for time; on drawing omitted the right arm of a figure; apathetic; convulsion after disappearance of denial

142

TABLE 2
CLINICAL, NEUROLOGICAL, PATHOLOGICAL AND BEHAVIORAL DATA IN CASES WITH IMPLICIT FORMS OF DENIAL

Case No., Sex, Age	Lesion	Neurological Findings	Spinal Fluid	Electroencephalogram	Behavior
53 F 24	Bifrontal meningioma; craniotomy	Papilledema; bilateral hyposmia; incontinence of urine and feces	Not done	Slow activity from 1 per sec. in both frontal regions and over left central region with superimposed bursts of 3 per sec. activity	Marked alteration in sexual behavior; paranoid, hypomanic; disorientation for time and place; melodramatic behavior; paraphasia; delusion of having a baby
54 M 49	Probable tumor of third ventricle; pneumoencephalogram showed filling defect in third ventricle with displacement of the iter and dilatation of both lateral ventricles and third ventricle shifted to right	Diminished vision bilaterally; incontinence of urine	Normal	Diffuse 4-6 per sec. activity, most marked over the frontal regions	Hypomanic, euphoric, paranoid; alteration in sexual behavior; reduplication for place; disorientation for time and place; ludic; paraphasia
55 F 34	Brain tumor unverified; pneumoencephalogram showed dis-	Left hemiparesis; left homonymous hemianopia; left hemi-	Not done	Diffuse bilateral delta activity from 1 to 6	Euphoric, paranoid, depressed, withdrawn; reduplication for place and time;

TABLE 2. (Continued)

Case No., Sex, Age	Lesion	Neurological Findings	Spinal Fluid	Electroencephalo-gram	Behavior
	tortion of third and lateral ventricles suggesting thalamic mass; sub-temporal decompression	anesthesia; incontinence of urine		per sec.	disorientation for time; confabulated journey; altered sexual behavior; tragic, dramatic manner; delusion that mother was alive; "hysterical" hemisensory syndrome; paraphasia
56 F 40	Right parietal infiltrating tumor (unverified); craniotomy; pneumoencephalogram and ventriculogram showed shift of ventricular system to left	Left hemiplegia; left-sided sensory loss; left-sided visual field defect; bilateral papilledema	Not done	1-3 per sec. slow activity at right frontal and temporal and ear lobe electrodes	Head and eyes averted to right; graphic denial; pain asymbolia; lethargic, depressed; disorientation for time and place
57 M 33	Glioblastoma right temporal lobe; craniotomy	History of headache, vomiting; left Babinski; left homonymous superior quadrantic visual field defect	Clear fluid; pressure 280 mm. of water; protein 39 mg./100 cc.	Irregular delta activity as low as 1 per sec., maximal at right ear lobe and anterior temporal electrodes, less at others	Euphoric, then depressed, lethargic; temporal reduplication; paraphasia; misidentification of persons
58 F	Hypertensive encephalopathy (?)	History of headaches; mental confusion	Clear; normal pressure; protein	Diffuse bilateral 3-6 per sec. slow	Reduplication for person and time; disorientation for

			15 mg./100 cc.	wave activity	
60					time and place; paranoid, depressed; hallucinations; paraphasia
59 F 17	Medulloblastoma; marked dilation of entire ventricular system; craniotomy; autopsy	Bilateral optic atrophy; ataxia of all limbs; nystagmus on lateral gaze; incontinence of urine and feces	Not done	Diffuse delta activity with frequencies from 1.5 per sec. bilaterally	Disorientation for time and place; euphoric, then depressed; noisy, demanding
60 M 59	Metastatic carcinoma of brain; carcinoma of lung; sub-temporal decompression	Left hemiplegia; incontinence of urine	Not done	Diffuse, bilateral non-symmetrical 4-6 per sec. activity	Withdrawal, depressed; disorientation for place; paraphasia
61 M 69	Glioblastoma in right frontotemporal region; craniotomy	Left hemiparesis; impaired spot-finding left hand	Clear; pressure 140 mm. of water; total protein 50 mg./100 cc.	Not done	Transient denial of operation; disorientation for time; clinging, childish; exposure
62 F 67	Subfrontal meningioma compressing right optic nerve; craniotomy; autopsy	History of convulsions; blindness and optic atrophy in O.D.; right pupil fixed to light	Clear fluid; normal pressure; total protein 94 mg./100 cc.	Bitemporal 1-2 per sec. activity with diffuse 4-6 per sec.	Euphoric, depressed; markedly facetious; reduplication for place and time; disorientation for place; hallucinations; paraphasia; sexual delusions
63 M 48	Gliogenous tumor in right temporo-parietal region; craniotomy	Left hemiparesis; left "hemianesthesia"; left homonymous hemianopia; papilledema	Not done	Diffuse delta activity as slow as 1 per sec. over entire right side; superimposed symmetrical diffuse	Marked withdrawal; depression; pain asymbolia; disorientation for time

TABLE 2. *(Continued)*

Case No., Sex, Age	Lesion	Neurological Findings	Spinal Fluid	Electroencephalogram	Behavior
				bursts of 2.5-4 per sec.	
64 M 29	Cerebellar astrocytoma; craniotomy; meningo-encephalitis	Papilledema; ataxic gait; incontinence of urine	Clear; 1000-2000 wbc	2-3 per sec. activity at posterior electrodes	Reduplication of body parts (head); reduplication for place and time; euphoric, paranoid; altered sexual behavior; ludic aspects; paraphasia
65 M 35	Glioblastoma right temporo-parietal region; autopsy	History of psychomotor convulsions; slight papilledema	Clear; normal pressure; protein 82 mg./100 cc.	Not recorded	Mild facetiousness; depression
66 M 28	Glioblastoma invading right parietal region; craniotomy	Blindness; papilledema; left hemiplegia and sensory loss; clonic jerking of left limbs; incontinence of urine and feces	Clear; pressure 130 mm. of water; total protein 68 mg./100 cc.	Diffuse 4-6 per sec. activity in all right leads	Transient denial of hemiplegia; disorientation for time and place; affable, calm, lethargic; acts as if he sees but admits blindness; delusion that father is alive; denial of having feeble-minded sister; reduplication for place
67 M 40	Glioblastoma invading right frontal lobe; craniotomy	Papilledema; left hemiparesis; incontinence of urine	Not done	Diffuse slow 3-6 per sec. activity in frontal and right parieto-temporal leads	Lethargic, restless, drowsy; paranoid; disorientation for place and time; reduplication for place and time

	Diagnosis; operation	Clinical findings	CSF	EEG	Mental status
68 F 33	Chromophobe pituitary adenoma; craniotomy	Bilateral optic atrophy; marked visual loss in O.D.; large central scotoma in O.S.; amenorrhea; incontinence of urine	Not done	Slow 1-3 per sec. activity over entire left hemisphere, most marked in temporo-parietal area	Apathetic, placid; disorientation for place and time; paraphasia; misidentification of people
69 F 25	Gunshot wound through right temporal region; craniotomy with evacuation of hematoma	Blindness and optic atrophy in O.D.; incontinence of urine	Not done	Not recorded	Bland, affable; disorientation for place and time; reduplication for place, time and person; paraphasia; delusion that mother was dead and that another girl was shot; confabulation of college degree and being pregnant and that brother was a Prisoner of War
70 M 68	Head injury; trephination	Marked memory loss; weakness of right arm; nystagmus on lateral gaze	Clear; pressure 180 mm. of water; protein 51 mg/100 cc.; 270 rbc	Diffuse symmetrical 6 per sec. activity	Reduplication for place, time and person; disorientation for place and time; paraphasia; alternately euphoric and depressed; hallucinations
71 F 47	Meningioma, inferior aspect of right temporal lobe; herniation of cerebellar tonsils; brain stem hemorrhages; craniotomy; autopsy	Papilledema; left hemiparesis; incontinence of urine	Not done	Diffuse bilateral 1-2 per sec. activity more marked on right	Paraphasia; disregarded left upper extremity; reduplication for place; disorientation for place; restless, depressed, fearful, paranoid; exposure

TABLE 2. (Continued)

Case No., Sex, Age	Lesion	Neurological Findings	Spinal Fluid	Electroencephalogram	Behavior
72 M 28	Pinealoma; skull x-ray showed calcifications in region of calcified pineal; ventriculogram showed mass projecting into third ventricle; craniotomy	Paralysis of upward gaze	Clear; pressure 160 mm. of water; total protein 41 mg./100 cc.; 36 lymphocytes	Low voltage slow 2-5 per sec. sporadic activity at posterior electrodes bilaterally	Reduplication for place and time; euphoric, paranoid; disorientation for time; paraphasia
73 M 60	Oligodendroglioma right frontoparietal region; craniotomy	History of convulsions; paresis of left limbs; hypalgesia of left upper extremity	Not done	Not done	Humor; reduplication for time and place
74 M 53	Undiagnosed; ventriculogram showed dilatation of lateral and third ventricles	Marked memory loss; right hemiparesis; incontinence of urine and feces; gross perceptual disturbance on double simultaneous stimulation	Clear; pressure 150 mm. of water; protein 63 mg./100 cc.	Delta activity from 1.5 to 4 per sec. over left frontal, temporal, ear lobe electrodes and right frontal and anterior temporal electrodes	Avoided right side; disorientation for place; lethargic; pedantic, stilted language
75 F 51	Glioblastoma right parieto-frontal area; pneumoencephalogram showed depression of right lateral ventricle and shift of	Left hemiparesis; bilateral Babinski; incontinence of urine	Clear; pressure 190 mm. of water; total protein 21 mg./100 cc.	Irregular delta activity at right parietal, frontal and central electrodes, less on left	Graphic denial; disorientation for time; restless, demanding, paranoid; altered sexual behavior; hallucinations

	Diagnosis and procedure	Clinical findings	CSF findings	EEG findings	Mental status
	...ventricular system to left; craniotomy				
76 F 62	Sarcoma right temporo-parietal region; craniotomy	Bilateral papilledema; left hemiparesis and sensory loss; left homonymous hemianopia; topographical disorientation; incontinence of urine	Clear; pressure 160 mm. of water	1-2 per sec. activity at all right-sided electrodes; large amount of 6 per sec. activity from all leads	Depressed, withdrawn; disorientation for place and time; paranoid; disregard for objects on left side
77 M 62	Head injury with subarachnoid bleeding; fracture through right parieto-occipital region	Bilateral papilledema and hemorrhage; incontinence of urine	Xanthochromic; pressure 330 mm. of water; total protein 190 mg./100 cc.	Symmetrical bursts of 3-5 per sec. activity at all leads	Disorientation for place and time; reduplication for place; restless, noisy; euphoric joking; hallucinations; paraphasia
78 M 56	Third ventricle tumor; pneumoencephalogram showed defect in posterior part of third ventricle; dilatation of anterior part and lateral ventricles; Torkildsen procedure	Ataxic gait; slurred speech; history of memory loss	Clear; pressure 110 mm. of water; protein 30 mg./100 cc.	Irregular 3-6 per sec. activity at left anterior temporal and ear lobe electrodes; symmetrical diffuse bursts of 2-3 per sec. activity	Lethargic, withdrawn; disorientation for place
79 F 58	Glioblastoma right fronto-parietal region; pneumoencephalogram revealed shift of ventricular system to left; craniotomy	Shuffling gait; marked bradykinesia	Clear; pressure 115 mm. of water; protein 165 mg./100 cc.	Diffuse 4-6 per sec. activity with bursts	Disorientation for place and time; lethargic, withdrawn; paraphasia; depressed

TABLE 2. (Continued)

Case No., Sex, Age	Lesion	Neurological Findings	Spinal Fluid	Electroencephalogram	Behavior
80 F 63	Subarachnoid hemorrhage probably on arteriosclerotic basis	History of convulsions; nystagmus on lateral and upward gaze; dysphasia	Bloody, then xanthochromic fluid	Diffuse and symmetrical 6 per sec. activity	Evasive answering questions about illness; reduplication for place; disorientation for place and time; drowsy, withdrawn, paranoid; sexual delusions; paraphasia
81 M 51	Third ventricle tumor (pinealoma?); ventriculogram showed large defect in third ventricle, dilatation of lateral ventricles; Torkildsen procedure	History of memory loss and convulsions; ataxic gait	Clear; pressure 190 mm. of water; protein 29 mg./100 cc.	Diffuse non-symmetrical 3-6 per sec. activity	Disorientation; reduplication for place and time; sometimes paranoid, lethargic; evasive when talking about illness; paraphasia
82 M 60	Squamous cell carcinoma of ethmoid with probable intracranial metastases	Papilledema with hemorrhages; hypalgesia right upper extremity	Clear; pressure 190 mm. of water; protein 60 mg./100 cc.	Diffuse 1-4 per sec. activity at both frontal and temporal electrodes	Reduplication for place and time; disorientation for place; evasive, withdrawal reaction when asked about illness; manneristic, lethargic, depressed, paranoid, ludic; paraphasia; altered sexual behavior
83 F	Subfrontal meningioma originating from	History of convulsions; left hemipar-	Xanthochromic; pressure 270 mm.	Slow 4-5 per sec. diffuse activity	Turned head and eyes to right; bland mood usually;

150

	Lesion / Procedure	Clinical findings	CSF	EEG	Mental status
50	tuberculum sellae; craniotomy and right frontal lobectomy	esis postoperatively; incontinence of urine	of water; total protein 32 mg./100 cc.	with bursts of 1-2 per sec. over frontal and temporal regions	paranoid sexual delusions; disorientation for time
84 F 43	Bilateral olfactory groove meningioma; craniotomy and right frontal lobectomy	Bilateral anosmia and optic atrophy	Xanthochromic fluid; pressure 160 mm. of water; total protein 46 mg./100 cc. (postoperatively)	Symmetrical bursts of 3-6 per sec. activity at frontal, temporal, ear lobe electrodes (preoperative)	Disorientation for place; misidentification of examiner; euphoric joking, later depressed and paranoid; hallucinations; paraphasia
85 F 59	Third ventricle tumor; ventriculogram showed lesion in posterior part of third ventricle, dilatation of anterior part and lateral ventricles; Torkildsen procedure	Weakness of lower extremities; right Babinski; marche à petit pas; incontinence of urine and feces	Clear fluid; pressure 170 mm. of water; protein 30 mg./100 cc.	Diffuse symmetrical 4-6 per sec. activity	Disorientation for place and time; euphoric, facetious; paranoid, irritable, depressed; altered sexual behavior
86 F 46	Subarachnoid hemorrhage; right carotid arteriogram showed small berry aneurysm at juncture of carotid and middle cerebral arteries	Stiff neck, eyeball tenderness	Bloody, then xanthochromic	Diffuse symmetrical 6 per sec. activity	Disorientation for place and time; euphoric and paranoid; restless, sleepy; altered sexual behavior; temporal reduplication
87 M 52	Bilateral olfactory groove meningioma; craniotomy and left	Bilateral anosmia; optic atrophy and almost complete visual	Not permitted by patient	Diffuse 1-3 per sec. activity, maximal at frontal and	Reduplication for time and person; disorientation for place and time; paranoid,

TABLE 2. (Continued)

Case No. Sex, Age	Lesion	Neurological Findings	Spinal Fluid	Electroencephalogram	Behavior
	frontal lobectomy	loss in O.S.		temporal leads	Irascible, euphoric, depressed, ludic; altered sexual behavior; paraphasia
88 F 47	Cerebro-vascular lesion; rheumatic heart disease	Left hemiparesis; left homonymous field defect; left-sided sensory loss; incontinence of urine	Clear; normal pressure	Diffuse slow wave activity as low as 0.6 per sec., more marked on right side	Hypomanic, much humor, altered sexual behavior; disorientation for time and place; head and eyes deviated to the right; graphic denial; paraphasia; hallucinations
89 M 56	Metastatic squamous cell carcinoma, left occipito-parietal area; craniotomy	Bilateral papilledema; right-sided sensory loss; right homonymous hemianopia; right Babinski; dyspraxia; dyspraxia; topographical disorientation; history of convulsions	Not done	Large amount of slow wave activity from 1.5 per sec. over entire left side; superimposed symmetrical bursts bilaterally	Transient denial of operation; disorientation for time and place; lethargic, depressed
90 M 48	Cerebro-vascular lesion; previous myocardial infarction and hypertension	Left hemiparesis; left astereognosis and sensory loss	Clear; normal pressure; protein 59 mg./100 cc.	Diffuse 1-3 per sec. activity at right electrodes; 4-5 per sec. activity bilaterally	Complete analgesia of left limbs; reduplication for person; disorientation for time of day; evasive, withdrawn, depressed, paranoid delusions; paraphasia

	Diagnosis	Neurological findings	CSF	EEG	Clinical symptoms
91 M 41	Ependymoma of third ventricle; craniotomy	Incontinence of urine	Not done	Diffuse bilateral 4-6 per sec. activity	Transient disorientation for time; withdrawn, depressed; hallucinations
92 M 54	Parieto-temporal gliogenous neoplasm, unverified; right carotid arteriogram showed elevation of middle cerebral vessel; craniotomy	Left hemiparesis, sensory loss; left homonymous hemianopia; incontinence of urine	Clear; pressure 180 mm. of water; total protein 87 mg./100 cc.	Diffuse slow activity, most marked in right temporoparietal region	Neglects left side of body; "hemianalgesia"; graphic denial; lethargic, paranoid, restless; rambling incoherent speech in response to questions about illness; disorientation for place and time; reduplication for place and time; marked withdrawal; paraphasia
93 M 47	Central nervous system lues	Weakness left lower extremity; absent KJ's and AJ's	Clear; 4 + Wasserman; pressure 160 mm. of water; 8 wbc; total protein 124 mg./100 cc.	Diffuse bursts of 4-6 per sec. activity	Paraphasia; pain asymbolia; reduplication for place and time; disorientation for place; vacuous, withdrawn
94 M 60	Probable cerebral embolus; rheumatic mitral stenosis	Right hemiplegia; right sensory loss; right homonymous hemianopia; dysphasia; incontinence of urine and feces	Slightly xanthochromic; 700 rbc; 300 wbc; total protein 206 mg./100 cc.	2.5 per sec. activity over entire left hemisphere; bilateral synchronous bursts	Neglect of right side; hemianesthesia of right side; graphic denial; head and eyes deviated to left; disorientation for time and place; restless; altered sexual behavior
95 F 50	Sarcoma of splenium of corpus callosum; craniotomy; autopsy	Papilledema and hemorrhages; incontinence of urine	Xanthochromic; pressure 240 mm. of water; total protein 150 mg./100 cc.	2-6 per sec. activity at right temporal, occipital, ear lobe and left ear lobe electrodes	Graphic denial; temporal reduplication; disorientation for place; euphoric, depressed, paranoid; altered sexual behavior; paraphasia

TABLE 2. (Continued)

Case No., Sex, Age	Lesion	Neurological Findings	Spinal Fluid	Electroencephalogram	Behavior
96 M 73	Encephalopathy of arteriosclerotic origin; pneumoencephalogram showed dilatation of third and lateral ventricles	Left homonymous hemianopia; left-sided hypesthesia demonstrable on double simultaneous stimulation; dyscalculia; dyspraxia; incontinence of urine	Xanthochromic fluid; pressure 170 mm. of water; total protein 192 mg./100 cc.	Large amount of 1-2 per sec. activity over right temporal region, less at right frontal, central and left temporal electrodes	Reduplication for place, time and person; disorientation for place and time; euphoric, depressed; comic ludic; paraphasia
97 M 48	Metastasis to right fronto-parietal region of carcinoma of breast; craniotomy	Papilledema; slight left hemiparesis; dyspraxia for dressing; finger dysgnosia; dyscalculia; incontinence of urine	Not done	Diffuse slow wave activity as low as 1 per sec. at right frontal, parietal, ear lobe and left frontal and inferior frontal electrodes; superimposed symmetrical bursts of 2-3 per sec. activity	Pain asymbolia; ignored left side of space; graphic denial; disorientation for place and time; lethargic, drowsy; paraphasia
98 M 34	Intracerebral hematoma, left fronto-parieto-temporal region; craniotomy	Right hemiparesis; dysphasia; right-sided sensory loss; incontinence of urine	Xanthochromic; pressure 300 mm. of water; total protein 155 mg./100 cc.	Diffuse slow wave 2-4 per sec. activity, diffuse on left and at right temporal, ear lobe and occipital electrodes	Avoids looking to right; pain asymbolia; temporal reduplication; disorientation for place and time; euphoric; paraphasia

	Diagnosis	Neurological signs	Cerebrospinal fluid	Electroencephalogram	Mental and behavioral findings
99 F 47	Subarachnoid hemorrhage; left carotid arteriogram normal	Left sixth nerve paralysis	Bloody; pressure 180 mm. of water	Not done	Reduplication for time; euphoric; altered sexual behavior; paraphasia
100 M 45	Subarachnoid hemorrhage; arteriogram normal	Right hemiparesis; incontinence of urine	Xanthochromic; pressure 100 mm. of water; protein 56 mg./100 cc.	Symmetrical low voltage fast activity	Evasive, jocular; disorientation for time and place; reduplication for person and time; sexual delusions; paranoid, agitated; paraphasia
101 M 62	Squamous cell carcinoma of lung with metastases to cerebellum; craniotomy	Papilledema; left Babinski; ataxia of left upper extremity	Slightly xanthochromic; pressure 130 mm. of water; total protein 104 mg./100 cc.	Normal preoperatively	Reduplication for place; disorientation for place and time; paraphasia; euphoric and depressed
102 F 36	Subarachnoid hemorrhage; left carotid angiogram showed arterial venous malformation involving vein of Galen; carotid ligation	Neck rigidity; bilateral Babinski; retinal hemorrhage	Xanthochromic; pressure 80 mm. of water; protein 49 mg./100 cc.	Normal	Reduplication for time and place; disorientation for place; euphoric, depressed; paraphasia
103 F 62	Undiagnosed disease of brain; pneumoencephalogram showed dilatation of right lateral and third ventricles; arteriogram showed no filling of suprasyl-	Left hemiplegia; left homonymous hemianopia; left-sided sensory loss; incontinence of urine and feces	Clear fluid; pressure 140 mm. of water; protein 84 mg./100 cc.	Slow wave activity as low as 1.2 per sec. at all electrodes, mainly right frontal	Ignored left side; graphic denial; temporal reduplication; disorientation for time and place; euphoric, paranoid; theatrical ludic behavior; altered sexual behavior; hallucinations; paraphasia

TABLE 2. (Continued)

Case No., Sex, Age	Lesion	Neurological Findings	Spinal Fluid	Electroencephalogram	Behavior
	vian branches of right middle cerebral artery				
104 M 51	Right thalamic tumor unverified; right carotid arteriogram showed displacement of veins in region of foramen of Monro	Left hemiparesis; left homonymous hemianopia; left dystereognosis	Not done	Diffuse 1.5-3.5 per sec. activity bilaterally, more on right	Avoided looking to left; reduplication for person; disorientation for place and time; clinging, demanding; paranoid, depressed, somewhat euphoric, withdrawn; hallucinations

REFERENCES

Albrecht, O.: Drei Fälle mit Antons Symptom. *Arch. f. Psychiat.*, 59:883-941, 1918.

Anton, G.: Blindheit nach beiderseitiger Gehirnerkrankung mit Verlust der Orientierung in Raume. *Mittherlungen des Vereines der Arzte in Steiermark*, 33:41-46, 1896.

Anton, G.: Ueber Herderkrankungen des Gehirnes, welche von Patienten selbst nicht wahrgenommen werden. *Wien. Klin. Wchnschr.*, 11:227-229, 1898.

Babinski, J.: Contribution à l'Etude des Troubles Mentaux dans l'Hémiplégie Organique Cérébrale (Anosognosie). *Rev. Neurol.*, 27:845-847, 1914.

Babinski, J.: Anosognosie. *Rev. Neurol.*, 25:365-366, 1918.

Babinski, J. and Joltrain, E.: Un nouveau cas d'anosognosie. *Rev. Neurol.*, 31:638-640, 1924.

Bechterev, V. M.: *Obozr. Psikhiat. i Nevrol.*, 1926. Cited by Schenderov and Gamaleja.

Bender, L.: Psychoses Associated with Somatic Diseases that Distort the Body Structure. *Arch. Neurol. & Psychiat.*, 32:1000-1029, 1934.

Bonhoeffer, K.: Casuistische Beiträge zur Aphasielehre. *Arch. f. Psychiat.*, 37:564-597, 1903.

Brockman, N. W. and Von Hagen, K. O.: Denial of Own Blindness (Anton's Syndrome): Report of Two Cases, One with Autopsy. *Bull. L. A. Neurol. Soc.*, 11:178-180, 1946.

Cairns, H., Oldfield, R. C., Pennybacker, J. B. and Whitteridge, D.: Akinetic Mutism with an Epidermoid Cyst of the Third Ventricle. *Brain*, 64:273-290, 1941.

Cobb, S.: Amnesia for the Left Limbs Developing into Anosognosia. *Bull. L. A. Neurol. Soc.*, 12:48-52, 1947.

Critchley, M.: A phantom supernumerary limb after a cervical root lesion. *Arq. Neuro-Psiquiat.*, 10:269-275, 1952.

Critchley, M.: *The Parietal Lobes.* London, Edward Arnold & Co., 1953.

Dejerine, J. and Vialet: Sur un cas de cécité corticale. *Compt. rend. Soc. de biol.*, 11:983-997, 1893.

Ehrenwald, H.: Verändertes Erleben des Körperbildes mit konsekutiver Wahnbildung bei linksseitiger Hemiplegie. *Mschr. Psychiat. Neurol.*, 75:89-97, 1930.

Fink, M. and Bender, M. B.: Development of Perception of Simultaneous Tactile Stimuli in Normal Children. *Neurology*, 3:27-34, 1953.

157

Fulton, J. F. and Bailey, P.: Tumors in the Region of the Third Ventricle: Their Diagnosis and Relation to Pathological Sleep. *J. Nerv. & Ment. Dis.*, 69:1-25, 145-164, 261, 1929.

Gerstmann, J.: Problem of Imperception of Disease and of Impaired Body Territories with Organic Lesions: Relation to Body Scheme and Its Disorders. *Arch. Neurol. & Psychiat.*, 48:890-913, 1942.

Goldstein, K.: *The Organism:* A Holistic Approach to Biology Derived from Pathological Data on Man. New York, American Book Co., 1939.

Guthrie, T. C. and Grossman, E. M.: A Study of the Syndromes of Denial. A.M.A., *Arch. Neurol. & Psychiat.*, 68:362-371, 1952.

Halloran, P. M.: Delusion of Body Scheme Due to Subdural Hematoma. *Bull. L. A. Neurol. Soc.*, 11:88-89, 1946.

Hamburg, D. A., Hamburg, B. and diGoza, S.: Adaptive Problems and Mechanisms in Severely Burned Patients. *Psychiatry*, 16:1-20, 1953.

Head, H. and Holmes, G.: Sensory Disturbances from Cerebral Lesions. *Brain*, 34:102-254, 1911.

Head, H.: *Aphasia and Kindred Disorders of Speech.* Cambridge, Cambridge University Press, 1926.

Isbell, H., Altschul, S., Kornetsky, C. H., Eisenman, A. J., Flanary, H. G. and Fraser, H. F.: Chronic Barbiturate Intoxication. *Arch. Neurol. & Psychiat.*, 64:1-28, 1950.

Ives, E. R. and Nielsen, J. M.: Disturbance of Body Scheme: Delusion of Absence of Part of Body in Two Cases with Autopsy Verification of the Lesions. *Bull. L. A. Neurol. Soc.*, 2:120-125, 1937.

Jackson, J. H.: *Selected Writings.* London, Hodder & Stoughton, 1932.

Kahn, R. L. and Schlesinger, B.: Preoperative and Postoperative Personality Changes Accompanying Frontal Lobe Meningioma. *J. Nerv. & Ment. Dis.*, 114:492-510, 1951.

Lejonne, P., Raymond, F. and Galezowski, J.: Cécité Corticale par Double Hemianopie. *Rev. Neurol.*, 19:680-691, 1906.

Lhermitte, J. and Garand: De l'anosognosie des Amputés. *Bull. Acad. Nat. Méd.*, 134:255-260, 1950.

Lunz, C.: Zwei Fälle von Korticaler Seelenblindheit. *Deutsche Med. Wchnschr.*, 1:381-393, 1897.

Lutt, C. J.: Denial of Blindness and Argyll-Robertson pupils without Syphilis. *Bull. L. A. Neurol. Soc.*, 12:189-191, 1947.

Mayer, C.: Eine doppelseitige homonyme Hemianopie mit Orientierungstörungen. *Mntschr. f. Psychiat. u. Neurol.*, 8:440-462, 1900.

Meerovich, R. I.: *Disturbance of the "Body Scheme" in Psychiatric Diseases.* Leningrad, Ministry of Public Health USSR, 1948.

Nathanson, M., Bergman, P. S. and Gordon, G. G.: Denial of Illness: Its Occurrence in One Hundred Consecutive Cases of Hemiplegia. *Arch. Neurol. & Psychiat.*, 68:380-387, 1952.

Nielsen, J. M. and Ives, E. R.: Generalized Autotopagnosia Due to Focal Cerebral Lesion: Its Resemblance to Finger-Agnosia, Disturbances of

Right and Left and Anosognosia of Babinski. *Bull. L. A. Neurol. Soc.*, 2:155-163, 1937.

Nielsen, J. M.: Gerstmann Syndrome: Finger Agnosia, Agraphia, Confusion of Right and Left and Acalculia: Comparison of this Syndrome with Disturbances of Body Scheme Resulting from Lesions of the Right Side of the Brain. *Arch. Neurol. & Psychiat.*, 39:536-560, 1938.

Nielsen, J. M. and Raney, R. B.: Symptomatology of Tumors of the Third Ventricle. *Bull. L. A. Neurol. Soc.*, 4:1-7, 1939.

Nielsen, J. M. and Sult, C. W.: Agnosias and the Body Scheme: Five Clinical Cases. *Bull. L. A. Neurol. Soc.*, 4:69-76, 1939.

Noble, D., Price, D. B., Gilder, R.: Psychiatric Disturbances following Amputation. *Am. J. Psychiat.*, 110:609-613, 1954.

Olsen, C. W. and Ruby, C.: Anosognosia and Autotopagnosia. *Arch. Neurol. & Psychiat.*, 39:536-560, 1938.

Oppenheimer, J. and Weissman, M.: On Anosognosia. *Am. J. Psychiat.*, 108:337-342, 1951.

Paterson, A. and Zangwill, O. L.: Recovery of Spatial Orientation in the Post-Traumatic Confusional State. *Brain*, 67:54-68, 1944.

Penfield, W. and Jasper, A.: *Epilepsy and the Functional Anatomy of the Human Brain.* Boston, Little Brown and Co., 1954.

Piaget, J.: *Play, Dreams and Imitation in Childhood.* New York, W. W. Norton and Co., 1951.

Pick, A.: On Reduplicative Paramnesia. *Brain*, 26:260-267, 1903.

Pick, A.: Ueber Störungen der Orientierung am eigenen Körper, in Arbeiten aus der psychiatrischen. *Klin. Prag.*, I: Berlin, Karger 1908.

Poetzl, O.: Ueber Störungen der Selbstwahrnehmung bei linkseitiger Hemiplegia. *Ztschr. f. d. ges. Neurol. u. Psychiat.*, 93:117-168, 1924.

Probst, M.: Ueber einen Fall vollstandiger Rindenblindheit und vollstandiger Amnesie. *Mntschr. f. Psychiat. u. Neurol.*, 9:5-21, 1901.

Raney, A. A. and Nielsen, J. M.: Denial of Blindness (Anton's Syndrome): Two Clinical Cases. *Bull. L. A. Neurol. Soc.*, 7:150-151, 1942.

Redlich, E. and Bonvicini, G.: Ueber das Fehlen der Wahrnehmung der eigenen Blindheit bei Hirnkrankheiten. *Jahrb. f. Psychiat.*, 29:1-134, 1908.

Redlich, F. C. and Dorsey, J. F.: Denial of Blindness by Patients with Cerebral Disease. *Arch. Neurol. & Psychiat.*, 53:407-417, 1945.

Rosenbaum, M.: "Pentothal Sodium" as an Adjunct in Therapy of Anxiety Hysteria: Report of a Case. *Arch. Neurol. & Psychiat.*, 60:70-76, 1948.

Rossolimo, G.: Ueber Hemianopsie und einseitige Ophthalmoplegie vascularen ursprungs. *Neurol. Centrlbl.*, 15:626-637, 1896.

Roth, M.: Disorders of the Body Image Caused by Lesions of the Right Parietal Lobe. *Brain*, 72:89-111, 1949.

Roth, N.: Unusual Types of Anosognosia and their Relation to the Body Image. *J. Nerv. & Ment. Dis., 100*:35-43, 1944.

Sandifer, P. H.: Anosognosia and Disorders of Body Scheme. *Brain, 69*: 122-137, 1946.

Sapir, E.: *Symbolism, in Encyclopedia of the Social Sciences,* New York, The Macmillan Co., 1934.

Schenderov, L. A. and Gamaleja, K. N.: Peculiar Disturbance of Body Scheme in Hemiplegics (Pseudomelia). *J. Nevrol., Psikhiat. i. Psikhogig., 4*:361-372, 1935.

Schilder, P.: Localization of the Body Image (Postural Model of the Body). *A. Res. Nerv. & Ment. Dis., 13*:466-484, 1932.

Shmarian, A.: On the Question of the Psychophysiological Principles of Depersonalization. *Sovet. Nevropat., Psikhiat. i. Psikhogig., 3*:67-96, 1934.

Spillane, J. D.: Disturbances of the Body Scheme: Anosognosia and Finger Agnosia. *Lancet, 1*:42-44, 1942.

Stengel, E. and Steele, G. D. F.: Unawareness of Physical Disability (Anosognosia). *J. Ment. Sc., 92*:379-388, 1946.

Tunero, J.: Ein Fall mit Antons Symptom. *Psychiat. et Neurol. Japon., 41*:679-690, 1931.

Von Hagen, K. O. and Ives, E. R.: Anosognosia (Babinski), Imperception of Hemiplegia: Report of Six Cases, One with Autopsy. *Bull. L. A. Neurol. Soc., 2*:95-103, 1937.

Weber, F. P.: Agnosia of Hemiplegia and of Blindness after Cerebral Embolism. *Lancet, 1*:44-46, 1942.

Weinstein, E. A. and Kahn, R. L.: Syndrome of Anosognosia. *Arch. Neurol. & Psychiat., 64*:772-791, 1950.

Weinstein, E. A. and Kahn, R. L.: Patterns of Disorientation in Organic Brain Disease. *J. Neuropath. & Clin. Neurol., 1*:214-225, 1951.

Weinstein, E. A. and Kahn, R. L.: Nonaphasic Misnaming (Paraphasia) in Organic Brain Disease. A.M.A. *Arch. Neurol. & Psychiat., 67*:72-79, 1952.

Weinstein, E. A., Linn, L. and Kahn, R. L.: Psychosis During Electroshock Therapy: Its Relation to the Theory of Shock Therapy. *Am. J. Psychiat., 109*:22-26, 1952.

Weinstein, E. A., Kahn, R. L. and Sugarman, L. A.: Phenomenon of Reduplication. A.M.A., *Arch. Neurol. & Psychiat., 67*:808-814, 1952.

Weinstein, E. A. and Kahn, R. L.: Personality Factors in Denial of Illness. A.M.A., *Arch. Neurol. & Psychiat., 69*:355-367, 1953.

Weinstein, E. A., Kahn, R. L., Sugarman, L. A. and Linn, L.: Diagnostic Use of Amobarbital Sodium ("Amytal Sodium") in Brain Disease. *Am. J. Psychiat., 109*:889-894, 1953.

Weinstein, E. A., Kahn, R. L., Sugarman, L. A. and Malitz, S.: Serial Administration of the "Amytal Test" for Brain Disease: Its Diagnostic and Prognostic Value. A.M.A., *Arch. Neurol. & Psychiat.*, 71:217-226, 1954.

Weinstein, E. A., Kahn, R. L., Malitz, S. and Rozanski, J.: Delusional Reduplication of Parts of the Body. *Brain*, 77:45-60, 1954.

Weinstein, E. A. and Malitz, S.: Changes in Symbolic Expression with Amobarbital Sodium ("Amytal Sodium"). *Am. J. Psychiat.*, 3:198-206, 1954.

Weinstein, E. A., Kahn, R. L. and Sugarman, L. A.: Ludic Behavior in Patients with Brain Disease. *J. Hillside Hosp.*, 3:98-106, 1954.

Weinstein, E. A., Malitz, S. and Barker, W.: Denial of the Loss of a Limb. *J. Nerv. & Ment. Dis.*, 120:27-30, 1954.

Wikler, A. and Rasor, R. W.: Psychiatric Aspects of Drug Addiction. *Am. J. Med.*, 14:566-570, 1953.

INDEX